The Effective M   ⌐ıι of
Prostatic Cancer

The Effective Management of Prostatic Cancer

Edited by

D Michael A Wallace FRCS
*Chairman, Oncology Section of the British Association of Urological Surgeons
and Consultant Urological Surgeon, Department of Urology,
Queen Elizabeth Hospital, Birmingham, UK*

R Tim D Oliver FRCP
*Sir Joseph Maxwell Professor in Medical Oncology,
St Bartholomew's Hospital, London, UK*

Dan Ash FRCR FRCP
*Immediate Past Dean, Faculty of Clinical Oncology of The Royal College of Radiologists
and Consultant Clinical Oncologist, Cookridge Hospital, Leeds, UK*

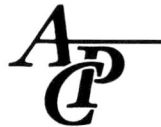

Andrew Miles MSc MPhil PhD
*Professor of Public Health Policy and UK Key Advances Series Organiser,
University of East London, UK*

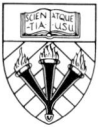

UeL University Centre for
Public Health Policy &
Health Services Research

Royal
College of
Radiologists

Association
of
Cancer Physicians

British Association
of Urological
Surgeons

AESCULAPIUS MEDICAL PRESS
LONDON SAN FRANCISCO SYDNEY

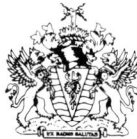

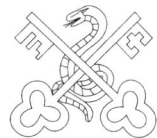

Published by

Aesculapius Medical Press (London, San Francisco, Sydney)
Centre for Public Health Policy and Health Services Research
School of Health Sciences
University of East London
PO Box LB48, London EC1A 1LB, UK

First published 2002

British Library Cataloguing in Publication Data
A catalogue record for this book is available from the British Library

ISBN 1 903044 25 1

While the advice and information in this book are believed to be true and accurate at the
time of going to press, neither the authors nor the publishers nor the sponsoring institutions
can accept any legal responsibility or liability for any errors or omissions that may be made.
In particular (but without limiting the generality of the preceding disclaimer) every effort
has been made to check drug usages; however, it is possible that errors have been missed.
Furthermore, dosage schedules are constantly being revised and new side effects recognised.
For these reasons, the reader is strongly urged to consult the drug companies' printed
instructions before administering any of the drugs recommended in this book.

Further copies of this volume are available from:

Claudio Melchiorri
Research Dissemination Fellow
Centre for Public Health Policy and Health Services Research
School of Health Sciences
University of East London
PO Box LB48, London EC1A 1LB, UK

Fax: 020 8525 8661
email: claudio@keyadvances4.demon.co.uk

Typeset, printed and bound in Britain
Peter Powell Origination & Print Limited

Contents

Contributors

Naomi E Allen DPhil, Research Fellow, Cancer Research UK Epidemiology Unit, University of Oxford

Wendy Ansell SRN, Macmillan Urology Nurse Specialist, St Bartholomew's Hospital, London

Dan Ash FRCR FRCP, Immediate Past Dean, Faculty of Clinical Oncology of The Royal College of Radiologists and Consultant Clinical Oncologist, Cookridge Hospital, Leeds

Frank Chinegwundoh FRCS FEBU, Consultant Urological Surgeon, St Bartholomew's Hospital, London

David P Dearnaley MA MD FRCP FRCR, Reader in Prostate Cancer Studies and Head of Urology Unit, Institute of Cancer Research and the Royal Marsden Hospital, London and Surrey

Douglas Easton PhD, Director, CRC Genetic Epidemiology Unit, Strangeways Research Laboratories, Cambridge

Rosalind A Eeles MA PhD FRCP FRCR, Team Leader, Translational Cancer Genetics Team, Institute of Cancer Research and Royal Marsden Hospital NHS Trust, London and Surrey

Mark R Feneley MD FRCS, Consultant Urologist, Nottingham City Hospital, Nottingham

Heather L Gould SRN, Macmillan Nurse Specialist, Southmead Hospital, Bristol

Michael Jarmulowicz FRCPath, Consultant Histopathologist, Royal Free Hospital, London

Amir V Kaisary MA ChM FRCS, Consultant Urological Surgeon, Royal Free Hospital, London

Timothy J Key PhD, Reader in Epidemiology, Cancer Research UK, Epidemiology Unit, University of Oxford

Ross Knight FRCS, Specialist Registrar in Urology, Royal Free Hospital, London

Tim Lane MB BS FRCS, Research Fellow in Uro-oncology, St Bartholomew's Hospital, London

Vinod Nargund PhD FRCS FEBU, Consultant Urological Surgeon & Honorary Senior Lecturer in Urology, St Bartholomew's Hospital, London

R Tim D Oliver FRCP, Sir Joseph Maxwell Professor in Medical Oncology, St Bartholomew's Hospital, London

Richard Parkinson MRCS, Research Fellow, Nottingham City Hospital, Nottingham

Anup Patel MS FRCS, Consultant Urological Surgeon, Department of Urology, St Mary's Hospital, London

Andreas Polychronis MB BCh MRCP, Specialist Registrar in Medical Oncology, St George's Hospital, London

Hugh S Rogers MB BChir FRCS, Consultant Urologist and Director for Modernisation, West Middlesex University Hospital, Middlesex

Edward Rowe MB BS, Clinical Research Fellow, Department of Urology, St Mary's Hospital, London

Robert Shearer FRCS (retired), Consultant Surgeon, Royal Marsden Hospital NHS Trust

Jyoti Shah MB BS, Clinical Research Fellow, Department of Urology, St Mary's Hospital, London

Rashmi Singh MB BS, Institute of Cancer Research, Sutton, Surrey

Paula Wells PhD MRCP FRCR, Consultant Medical Oncologist, St Bartholomew's Hospital, London

Preface

In Britain, around 20,000 men are diagnosed with prostate cancer and about 10,000 men die from the disease each year, making it the second most common carcinoma after lung cancer. The number of men diagnosed is increasing year on year, although it is important to recognise that this 'increase' may be explained in part by earlier diagnosis and the increased detection of non-aggressive cancers as a result of greater public awareness and more intensive medical investigation. Worldwide, prostate cancer rates are high in Westernised countries and low, but increasing, in most less developed countries.

Although the cause of prostate cancer has long been unclear, the modern view is that it, like lung cancer, is initiated in early puberty and develops over a 30- to 50-year life under the influence of androgens, as well as dietary, infectious and chemical/radiation exposures against a background of genetic susceptibility/resistance. About 5–10% of patients presenting with prostatic cancer demonstrate a family history of the disease. Recent studies indicate that such disposition is likely to be mediated through both highly penetrant and lower penetrance genes, with linkage studies having suggested multiple locations for high-risk prostate cancer genes, including chromosome 1q24 (*HPC1*), 1q42, 1p36 and Xq. A recent locus has also been suggested at 20q and other weaker suggestions of locations have also been described. No genetic cloning procedures were successfully completed until October 2000, at which time a gene located at 17p (*HCP2*) was successfully cloned with sequence variants identified which may be associated with a 2.7-fold prostate cancer risk.

Results from the CRC/BPG UK Familial Prostate Cancer Study and the ACTANE consortium have contributed much to the understanding of the genetic basis of prostate cancer. Indeed, ACTANE data have shown that *HPC1* is more likely to contribute to larger families; four cases and a meta-analysis of 772 families from a worldwide international consortium have shown that only about 6% of prostate cancer families are likely to be caused by *HPC1*. Indeed, overall, evidence is accumulating to suggest against linkage for Xq, 1p36 and 1q42 loci, and which indicates that the Xq gene is far more likely to be present in smaller clusters and 1p36 associated with earlier onset of disease, although not with any other cancers. Other associated studies have shown that approximately 5% of prostate cancer clusters may be the result of germline mutations in the breast cancer-predisposition gene *BRCA*-2, which has immediate implications for the screening of female relatives in such prostate cancer clusters; recent research has been directed at investigating precisely what percentage of young-onset cases are caused by *BRCA*-2. Importantly, studies of low-penetrance genes have shown that longer repeat lengths in the androgen receptor gene (16-GGC repeats) are associated with a halving of disease-free survival and have identified a genotype at increased risk (GST T/M null and GST P val/val) that is associated with a 1.8-fold risk. The observation that selenium may possess protective properties has led to studies that have aimed to assess an association of genotypes of the selenium-dependent glutathione enzyme (GPX) with prostate cancer risk. All such results may be useful in identifying individuals at increased risk of developing prostate cancer, with the aim of ensuring access to targeted screening and prevention. Part 1 of this text discusses all of these data in considerable detail and provides a stimulating review of our current knowledge of the epidemiology and genetics of the disease.

Part 2 is concerned with diagnosis, discussing the so-called 'window of opportunity' for curative intervention in terms of early diagnosis and the fast tracking of patients for appropriate interventions. Observational studies in men undergoing total prostatectomy as the treatment of choice for clinically organ-confined cancer indicate that the likelihood of microscopic metastases is significantly greater when the cancer is high grade or not pathologically organ confined. Thus, to achieve cure with definitive local treatment, it is axiomatic that early diagnosis should be aimed towards men most likely to have a cancer that is organ confined and the appropriate use of biochemical and histological markers is of considerable clinical utility in this context. Indeed, recent outcome analysis data from the Johns Hopkins hospital indicate that men with a prostate-specific antigen (PSA) level of < 12 ng/ml in whom biopsies show a Gleason Score of < 7 have an extremely high probability of long-term PSA-free survival after definitive local treatment. Biochemical recurrence is significantly greater in men with PSA levels > 12 ng/ml or Gleason Score > 7, but it does not necessarily preclude long-term metastasis-free survival. PSA testing offers a window of opportunity for detection of prostate cancer at a stage when surgical or radiotherapeutic treatment could be curative, although it also leads to an increase in diagnosis of latent disease, which may not be life threatening, as well as distressful investigation of patients with false-positive tests. The challenge for the next decade is threefold: first, to minimise this disadvantage by improved diagnostic tests, improved understanding of the natural history and medical management of the precursor lesions; second, to improve the techniques of treatment to minimise the complications; third, to develop prognostic indicators and modelling techniques based on progression rates for better identification of the appropriate time for multimodality intervention to take advantage of the improved toxicity profile of the improved treatment modalities.

It is well documented that delays routinely occur in access of the patient with cancer to appropriate treatment in the UK, but there is some evidence to suggest that these are now being modified through the national cancer collaborative programme, the aims of which are to improve the experience and outcomes for patients with suspected or diagnosed cancer. Nine sites across England, for example, are now working on five cancers, including cancer of the prostate, with the aim of implementing positive change through the use of a methodology involving process mapping to aid re-design, the pre-scheduling of steps in the journey (e.g. consultation and biopsy, results clinics, staging, treatment), the matching of capacity and demand to resolve so-called 'bottlenecks' in service provision, and the reduction in delays and the support of patients with relevant information when they want it. This approach has certainly been shown to be capable, in some of the institutions studied to date, of improving results. Indeed, electronic referral protocols and 'faxback' procedures can now give patients their appointment before leaving the GP's surgery, the time from referral to identification of patients at risk from prostate cancer can be reduced from 6 months to 2 weeks by a nurse-led clinic, pre-planning and booking can reduce waiting times, multidisciplinary patient records and patient-held results logs can be developed, and patient information leaflets can be tailored to events. All of these improvements and re-engineering of systems may usefully guide quality improvement initiatives in a majority of institutions, leading to measurable reductions in referral delay, improvements in access to specialist care and increases in patient satisfaction.

A detailed exposition of the scientific evidence and expert clinical opinion base underpinning surgical and medical intervention in established disease forms Part 3. Traditionally, surgical intervention has been widely considered as the preferred initial option and one that should aim at cure. A proper understanding of the significance of histological data, PSA level, clinical stage and Gleason Score has been of integral use in predicting the stage of localised prostatic carcinoma and in selecting the ideal patients for this particular modality of treatment. The impact of radical prostatectomy on patient welfare, quality of life, continency and sexual potency remain, however, central issues of major concern. Androgen ablation has been known to produce marked regression of prostate cancer for over half a century and interest in combined modality treatment for localised disease has recently increased, because of both the availability of reversible methods of androgen ablation and the development of PSA testing which, as discussed, has been shown to be a remarkably sensitive index of disease recurrence. Indeed, prostate cancer patients can now be identified as having a high risk of failing single modality treatment based on pre-treatment PSA levels, clinical stage and Gleason Score. In particular, a PSA of > 20 ng/ml predicts a biochemical failure rate of over 50% when monotherapies are given, and this has led to the development of treatment strategies that combine the modalities of external beam radiotherapy and neoadjuvant hormone treatment, particularly in localised disease. An additional therapy that has to date demonstrated remarkable results is brachytherapy and, although a major limitation of the study of the effectiveness of this technique has been the lack of randomised controlled trials comparing it with other treatments, fascinating data have been generated from several hundred patients over more than 5 years of follow-up. These data show that it is possible to identify a group of patients who do well with brachytherapy alone (i.e. PSA < 10, Gleason Score ≤ 6). These patients have a 70–80% probability of biochemical disease-free control at 10 years. Results are not so good for poorer prognosis patients and there remains some uncertainty about the role of external beam radiotherapy and hormone therapy in these groups. The quality of implantation is important in achieving both disease-free control and minimal morbidity. and quality indices have been identified to guide practice. The risk of incontinence is approximately 1% and the risk of impotence approximately 30%. For well-selected patients. brachytherapy provides a quick and simple treatment with high levels of biochemical control and very low levels of morbidity.

Part 4, the final section, is concerned with issues of clinical governance of prostate cancer services. The availability of specialist knowledge in the management of prostatic cancer and efficient relationships between cancer units and cancer centres in the provision and application of such knowledge are paramount considerations in the delivery of anything that could be called an 'effective' service. It is in this context that the pivotal role of the multidisciplinary clinical team becomes clear and an elegant description is given of the structure and functioning of the team, with a particular emphasis on the co-ordinating role of clinical nurse specialists and their role in the provision of appropriate information to patients. The comprehensive discussion of the effectiveness of given treatments for prostate cancer and their delivery within the context of the clinical service that forms the central core of the book would be incomplete without an accompanying consideration of the economic impact of prostate cancer and the costs associated with the provision of care. At the time of writing, the value of prostate cancer screening using PSA testing remains disputed and, furthermore, target populations for prostate cancer 'case detection' have still not been clearly defined, leading to wasted resources through indiscriminate testing in men unsuitable for curative therapy. To be sure, however, prostate cancer screening is undoubtedly more cost-effective than, say, mammographic screening is for breast cancer. Indeed, the benefits of early detection in high-prevalence groups may be thought highly likely to result in cost savings through avoidance of the costs ultimately generated by the treatment of advanced disease in these men.

Considerable variation in the costs and outcomes of care of men with cancer of the prostate continue to be documented within the literature and these appear to be the result of a multiplicity of factors that are enumerated and discussed with great clarity in the concluding work. Indeed, as the authors emphasise, the challenges of providing high-quality, cost-effective prostate cancer services involve the reliable detection of significant disease at a curable stage using a 'cheap' test that meets screening criteria, in providing a selection of curative local treatments with low morbidity that are attractive to patients and thus avoiding the high costs in terms of disease treatment and death that will otherwise be incurred. To meet these challenges in 2002 and beyond, we need to develop a national network of specialist reference centres supported by networks of referring urologists and oncologists where care can be provided by focused multidisciplinary teams of subspecialists and dedicated members of allied professions. It is really only in this setting that individual treatment outcomes will be optimised and the process of care made more efficient. The provisions of the NHS Cancer Plan go some way in addressing such concerns in relation to all cancer, that of the prostate included, although intention and action are not to be confused and a second edition of this volume, due in 2003, will report an evaluation of what might be termed 'operational progress against policy statements'.

In the current age, where doctors and health professionals are increasingly overwhelmed with clinical information, we have aimed to provide a fully current, fully referenced text that is as succinct as possible but as comprehensive as necessary. Consultants in urology, clinical and medical oncology and their trainees will find it of particular use as part of continuing professional development and specialist training respectively and we advance it as an excellent tool for these purposes. We anticipate, however, that the volume will also prove of considerable use to specialist nurses in urology and oncology as a valuable reference text and to the managers of cancer services as part of their own work and we commend the book enthusiastically to these colleagues for these purposes.

In conclusion, we thank AstraZeneca UK Ltd for a grant of educational sponsorship that helped organise a national conference held with the British Association of Urological Surgeons, The Royal College of Radiologists and the Association of Cancer Physicians at The Royal College of Pathologists, at which synopses of the constituent chapters of this book were presented.

Michael Wallace FRCS
Tim Oliver FRCP
Dan Ash FRCR
Andrew Miles MSc MPhil PhD

Acknowledgements

The following colleagues contributed as members of the expert planning committee for the year 2000/2001 prostate cancer UK key advances project: Mr John Anderson, Dr Dan Ash, Dr Roger Buchanan, Dr David Dearnaley, Professor Andrew Miles, Professor Tim Oliver and Mr Michael Wallace. The contribution of Dr Andreas Polychronis, Specialist Registrar in Medical Oncology, St. George's Hospital, London, as secretary to the committee and assistant editor in the preparation of the current volume, is also acknowledged.

PART 1

Genetics and epidemiology

Chapter 1

Genetic predisposition and environmental influences on the genesis of prostate cancer

Rashmi Singh, Rosalind A Eeles, Robert Shearer, Douglas Easton and the CRC/BPG UK Familial Prostate Cancer Study Collaborators and the UK Familial Prostate Cancer Study Coordination Group

Introduction

Prostate cancer is of significant international public health importance. From the statistics of 2000, approximately 13,000 cases had been diagnosed each year in England and Wales and prostate cancer causes approximately 10,000 deaths (Office for National Statistics 2000). In the USA, it is the most common malignancy in men, and over 180,000 new cases were projected to be diagnosed in 2000 (Landis *et al.* 1999). In Europe, the incidence is increasing by 10–20% every 5 years, even after accounting for the increase in numbers of prostate cancer cases identified through screening (Coleman *et al.* 1993).

The underlying causes for this disease are not fully known. Various risk factors (Dijkman & Debruyne 1996) have been proposed such as dietary, endocrine and sexually transmitted agents, but as yet none of these environmental factors has been confirmed as a significant cause of prostate cancer.

The prevalence of this disease varies markedly between different ethnic groups, with the highest frequency found in African–Americans and the lowest frequency in Asian populations (Parkin *et al.* 1993; Whittemore *et al.* 1995). The extent to which this ethnic disparity is attributable to environmental or genetic factors is unknown.

Epidemiological studies of prostate cancer have shown familial clustering of this disease and it is now well recognised that a positive family history of prostate cancer is a strong risk factor. Approximately 5–10% of patients are found to have a family history of the disease. This suggests the existence of underlying genetic predisposing factors and has led to attempts to map the gene or genes predisposing to prostate cancer by groups such as the CRC/BPG UK Familial Prostate Cancer Study. Although various chromosomal loci have been reported as sites for prostate cancer susceptibility genes, results have been conflicting and a gene still remains to be cloned.

Epidemiological evidence

Various case–control (Morganti & Aea 1956; Woolf 1960; Cannon 1982) and cohort studies, reviewed by Eeles (1999), have investigated the role of family history as a risk factor for prostate cancer development. Much evidence comes from population studies in Utah where large pedigrees with multiple cancer cases are found. In families with a positive history of prostate cancer in a first-degree relative (i.e. brother, father or son), these groups reported an overall threefold increased risk of the disease, with relative risk estimates ranging from 1.76 to 7.5. As seen in Table 1.1, risk is less but still significant if only a second-degree relative is affected (grandfather or uncle). Maximal elevation in risk, however, occurs if both first- and second-degree relatives are affected when the relative risk increases to 8.8 (Steinberg *et al.* 1990). Moreover, this relative risk increases as the number of affected members in the family increases (Table 1.2): having three first-degree relatives affected gives an 11-fold increased risk for developing prostate cancer (Steinberg *et al.* 1990).

Table 1.1 Relative risks for prostate cancer in relatives of prostate cancer cases by degree of relationship (from Steinberg *et al.* 1990)

Affected relatives	Relative risk (95%CI)
First degree	2.0 (1.2–3.3)
Second degree	1.7 (1.0–2.9)
Both first and second degree	8.8 (2.8–28.1)

95%CI, 95% confidence interval.

Table 1.2 Age-adjusted relative risk estimates for prostate cancer by number of additional affected family members (from Steinberg *et al.* 1990)

Affected relatives (besides proband)	Odds ratio (95%CI)
1	2.2 (1.4–3.5)
2	4.9 (2.0–12.3)
3	10.9 (2.7–43.1)

Early age at diagnosis of the proband was also found to be an important determinant of risk of prostate cancer to relatives. As shown in Table 1.3, the brother of a proband diagnosed with prostate cancer at age 50 has a relative risk of 1.9-fold of developing the disease compared with a brother of a case diagnosed at age 70 (Carter *et al.* 1992). The magnitude of the increased relative risk as the age of the proband decreases and the closeness and number of the affected family members increase cannot be explained by environmental factors alone, supporting a role for a genetic aetiology.

Twin studies also lend support to the existence of an underlying genetic predisposition to prostate cancer. Monozygotic twins have been found to have a fourfold increased concordance rate for the development of prostate cancer compared with dizygotic twins, confirming the importance of genetic factors (Grönberg *et al.* 1994).

Table 1.3 Estimated risk ratios for prostate cancer in first-degree relatives of probands, by age at onset in proband and additional family members (from Carter *et al.* 1992)

Age at onset of proband (years)	No additional relatives affected (95%CI)	One or more additional first-degree relatives affected (95%CI)
50	1.9 (1.2–2.8)	7.1 (3.7–13.6)
60	1.4 (1.1–1.7)	5.2 (3.1–8.7)
70	1.0[a]	3.8 (2.4–6.0)

[a]Reference group.

Segregation analyses

Segregation analysis involves studying the family aggregation of prostate cancer to determine the likely mode of inheritance and penetrance of prostate cancer susceptibility genes.

Several segregation analyses, performed on prostate cancer families (Carter *et al.* 1992), evaluated 690 families of radical prostatectomy patients. Their data suggested that inherited susceptibility to prostate cancer was the result of a rare, highly penetrant, autosomal dominant gene with a population frequency of 0.003. The cumulative risk of prostate cancer by the age of 85 was estimated to be 88% in carriers compared with only 5% in non-carriers. The gene accounted for approximately 43% of prostate cancer cases diagnosed under the age of 55 years and 9% of cases in total.

Two further segregation analyses by Grönberg *et al.* (1997a) and Schaid *et al.* (1998) (Table 1.4) also proposed similar transmission models. Although these three studies used different populations, they all produced consistent support for the presence of at least one highly penetrant, autosomal dominant, prostate cancer susceptibility gene. Traditionally such genes have been sought using linkage analysis of large pedigrees with multiple affected cases of the disease. This approach has been successfully applied to other common cancers such as melanoma (Cannon-Albright *et al.* 1992) and breast cancer (Hall *et al.* 1990; Wooster *et al.* 1994).

Linkage analysis

Based on the findings of these segregation analyses, the search for prostate cancer susceptibility genes commenced. High-risk prostate cancer families for study are selected according to different criteria by different groups. The CRC/UK Familial Prostate Cancer study has a multi-faceted approach to try to identify both the high and lower penetrance genes believed to be involved in this disease. Therefore

Table 1.4 Comparison of segregation analyses

	Carter et al. *(1992)*	Grönberg et al. *(1997a)*	Schaid et al. *(1998)*
No. of patients	691	2,600	4,288
Genetic model	AD*	AD	AD
Gene frequency (%)	0.3	1.7	0.6
Penetrance by age 85 (%)	88	63	89

All models' risk curves start to rise at 50 years.
AD, autosomal dominant.

collection of DNA is targeted at several groups. Families fulfilling one or more of the following criteria are selected for study (Eeles 1999):

- multiple-case prostate cancer families with three or more cases at any age;
- two or more affected relative pairs where one is under 65 years at diagnosis.

As a result of collaboration with Canada, Texas, Australia, Norway and EU Biomed (Italy Austria) to form the ACTANE Consortium, there are 194 such families for linkage studies.

DNA samples have also been collected from 285 single cases diagnosed with early onset prostate cancer (age 55 years or less). In addition we have a systematic series of over 1,000 prostate cancer patients treated at one centre.

Linkage studies involve genotyping affected individuals (and unaffected, only to infer genotypes of affected deceased individuals) from these informative families for genetic markers distributed across the genome, using either blood or tissue DNA. If one or more markers in a region are found to segregate with the disease trait within the family set, this suggests the presence of a potential susceptibility gene in this location. The LOD score is the logarithm of the odds of linkage and an LOD of >3.0 ($\log_{10} 3.0 = 1,000$ to 1 odds of linkage) is considered to be significant. An LOD of < –2.0 is evidence against linkage of 100 to 1.

Putative loci for prostate cancer genes

To date, four main chromosomal loci have emerged as candidate regions for prostate cancer genes and have been extensively studied by numerous international groups. In addition to these four loci, new evidence has emerged for *HPC2*, a prostate cancer gene that has recently been cloned on chromosome 17p.

HPC1: hereditary prostate cancer 1 gene (1q24-25)

In 1996, Smith *et al.* performed a genome-wide search with linkage analysis in 91 high-risk prostate cancer families. They reported linkage of prostate cancer to chromosome 1q24-25 and named the locus *HPC1*. The maximal multi-point LOD score was 5.43 under heterogeneity (as stated above, a LOD score of >3 is considered to be statistically significant). Interestingly, two of the linked families were African–American and contributed to over 1.00 of the total LOD score. Although the initial report of linkage to *HPC1* proposed that up to 34% of prostate cancer families could be linked to this locus, a subsequent pooled analysis of 772 families (Xu 2000a, 2000b) showed the actual proportion to be much lower at 6%. Following this first report of linkage, the UK/Canadian/Texan Linkage Consortium found negative evidence for linkage in the 1q24-25 region in 136 prostate cancer families; the estimated proportion of families linked was 4% with no evidence in families with less than three affected. However, up to 20% of families with four or more cases could have been linked to this locus (Eeles *et al.* 1998). This was the first study to suggest that *HPC1* may be more likely to be present in larger clusters. Subsequently, other studies have shown that families with male-to-male disease transmission, early age at diagnosis (65 years or less) and five or more affected members are more likely to be linked to chromosome 1q24-25 (Xu 2000a, 2000b).

Since the initial report by Smith *et al.* (1996) on *HPC1,* several groups have aimed to confirm these findings in their family sets. Four studies have shown only weak linkage to the locus using non-parametric methods (Cooney *et al.* 1997; Hsieh *et al.* 1997; Neuhausen *et al.* 1999; Berry *et al.* 2000a). In the study by Cooney *et al.* (1997), 6 of 59 families were African–American and again contributed disproportionately to the observation of linkage. Other studies, however, have failed to find evidence of linkage (McIndoe *et al.* 1997; Eeles *et al.* 1998; Bergthorsson *et al.* 2000; Goode *et al.* 2000a; Suarez *et al.* 2000a). In the large study by Goode *et al.* (2000), of 640 men from 150 high-risk prostate cancer families, linkage to multiple 1q24-25 markers was strongly rejected. Assuming heterogeneity, the estimated proportion of families linked (alpha) to *HPC1* in the entire dataset was only 2.6%.

Bergthorsson *et al.* (2000) also looked for allelic imbalance at *HPC1* to see if this gene may be acting as a tumour-suppressor gene. In tumours selected from their set of 87 Icelandic prostate cancer families, allelic imbalance was found in only 0–9%.

A similar low frequency of allelic imbalance at the *HPC1* locus was found by Ahman *et al.* (2000) in their study of 31 prostate tumours taken from Swedish men with hereditary prostate cancer.

A study of 33 potentially *HPC1*-linked families has indicated that *HPC1* is relatively site specific, although a moderate but not statistically significant excess of breast and colon cancer was found in the potentially *HPC1*-linked families compared with the unlinked families. The tumours in *HPC1* families tend to be higher grade and therefore would be expected to have a poorer prognosis, but this is not yet known (Grönberg *et al.* 1997b). Loss of heterozygosity studies by Dunsmuir *et al.* (1998) indicate that *HPC1* is very unlikely to be a tumour-suppressor gene.

The gene at the *HPC1* locus remains to be identified and indeed the localisation information is presently limited.

PCAP

A second putative prostate cancer susceptibility locus (*PCAP*) was reported by Berthon *et al.* (1998) at 1q42.2-43, a locus 60-cM downstream from *HPC1*.

This group estimated that as many as 40–50% of their French and German families could be linked to this locus. Again the evidence for linkage came predominantly from families with young onset cases (≤60 years). However, subsequent studies of the *PCAP* region by Gibbs *et al.* (1999a),Whittemore *et al.* (1999), Berry *et al.* (2000a), Bergthorsson *et al.* (2000) and Singh and the ACTANE Consortium (2000) have not found significant evidence of linkage, thus failing to confirm this locus. A replication linkage study by Suarez *et al.* (2000b) gave equivocal evidence for a prostate cancer susceptibility locus at chromosome 1q42.2-43. Therefore, although a small proportion of prostate cancer families may be linked to chromosome 1q42.2-43, it is likely to be considerably less than the 50% originally reported.

CAPB

In 1999, evidence for a third locus on chromosome 1 linked to familial prostate cancer was reported by (Gibbs *et al.* 1999b). This rare prostate cancer-brain cancer susceptibility locus, *CAPB,* at chromosome 1p36, was identified through linkage studies in 12 high-risk prostate cancer families with at least one family member with primary brain cancer. The overall LOD score in these families was 3.22, and after exclusion of 3 of the 12 families that had better evidence of linkage to other previously discussed prostate cancer susceptibility loci, a two-point LOD score of 4.74 was achieved. This group therefore concluded that a significant proportion of the families with both a high risk for prostate cancer and a family member with brain cancer showed linkage to the 1p36 region. However, the *CAPB* region was not subsequently confirmed by Berry *et al.* (2000a) in their report. The UK results do not find convincing evidence of linkage, although the LOD score is higher in families with younger average age of onset of prostate cancer. However, no correlation was found with tumours of any other primary site (Badzioch *et al.* 2001) unlike the first report.

Results of a linkage study in 149 prostate cancer families by Goode *et al.* (2000) suggested linkage to *CAPB* in patients with high-grade cancers, when clinical data were also incorporated into the analysis.

HPCX

In many case–control studies, the relative risk of prostate cancer has been higher for brothers than for fathers of men with the disease. In the study by Schaid *et al.* (1998) prostate cancer was 1.5 times more common among brothers than among the fathers of men with prostate cancer. These findings could be explained by an X-linked or recessive inheritance of prostate cancer susceptibility in some families. Indeed, in 1998, Xu *et al.* proposed a prostate cancer susceptibility locus on the long arm of chromosome X at Xq 27-28. Evidence for linkage was found in a combined study population of 360 North American, Swedish and Finnish families, with a peak two-point LOD score of 4.6. The estimated proportion of families linked to *HPCX* was 16%. To date there have been few follow-up reports attempting to confirm linkage of prostate cancer to *HPCX*. Within the UK set, we found no significant evidence of linkage overall, although the *Xq* gene may play a role in smaller clusters with the disease. Similarly Bergthorsson *et al.* (2000) found negative evidence for linkage at eight markers in the *HPCX* region. However, Lange *et al.* (1999) reported positive LOD scores over a 30-cM region containing *HPCX*, with the greatest evidence for linkage in the subset of families with no evidence of male-to-male transmission and early onset disease (<65 years).

There is currently much interest in this locus at Xq27-28 and it is anticipated that the HPCX gene may soon be cloned.

HPC2

HPC2/ELAC2 is a novel and recently cloned prostate cancer susceptibility gene on chromosome 17p. This gene was found to harbour mutations that segregate with prostate cancer in two high-risk pedigrees. In addition, two common mis-sense changes in the gene were found to be associated with prostate cancer. Survival analysis of cases carrying the mis-sense mutation Ala541Thr showed a significant decrease in length of survival compared with non-carrying cases in the pedigrees (Tavtigian *et al.* 2000).

Other candidate loci

Overall, the four proposed loci for high-penetrance prostate cancer genes mentioned above appear to account for only a minority of familial prostate cancer clusters and other putative genes have yet to be identified. Recent localisation of further prostate cancer susceptibility loci has emerged from genomic screens of large sets of prostate cancer families: a genome-wide search on 162 North American families with three or more members affected with prostate cancer has recently found evidence of linkage to a novel locus at chromosome 20q13, with a maximum two-point LOD score of 2.69, which is below statistical significance (Berry *et al.* 2000b). Interestingly, unlike *HPC1*, the strongest evidence of linkage was found in families with fewer than five affected relatives, a later average age of diagnosis and no male-to-male transmission. The results of another genome screen led by Suarez *et al.* (2000a) were also published recently. Their analysis of 504 brothers with prostate cancer identified five new regions of interest based on positive linkage signals: 2q, 12p, 15q, 16p and 16q. This last region, which was found to have the highest signal, has previously been reported as a candidate area for a tumour-suppressor gene in prostate cancer by Carter *et al.* (1990) and Bergerheim *et al.* (1991). Stratification of the sample population in the study by Suarez identified three further regions of interest: families with a history of breast cancer showed evidence of linkage to chromosome 1q35.1; those with no family history of prostate cancer had linkage to a region proximal to *HPC1* and those with late-onset disease had linkage at chromosome 4q.

Finally, a third genomic scan of 94 prostate cancer families by Gibbs *et al.* (2000) has proposed multiple regions of interest, including loci on chromosomes 10,12 and 14.

These new candidate loci for prostate cancer susceptibility genes reported from linkage studies have yet to be confirmed by other groups.

The role of *BRCA1* and *BRCA2*

Both breast and prostate cancer are hormone-dependent malignancies and epidemiological studies have shown a familial association between these two cancers (Thiessen 1974; Anderson & Badzioch 1992; Tulinius *et al.* 1992; Goldgar *et al.* 1994; Sellers *et al.* 1994).

Studies from the the Breast Cancer Linkage Consortium (1999) and by Ford *et al.* (1994) have suggested that male carriers of the *BRCA1* gene have a threefold increased risk of mortality from prostate cancer, whereas *BRCA2* carriers have a relative risk of prostate cancer of 4.65 (CI 3.48–6.22, $p < 0.0001$). The authors have assessed the overall contribution of the candidate genes *BRCA1* and *BRCA2* to familial prostate cancer by linkage analysis in a set of 100 multiple case families collected by the UK/Canadian part of the ACTANE Consortium. Neither locus showed significant evidence of linkage. The proportion of familial prostate cancer which may be due to either *BRCA1* or *BRCA2* was estimated to be 30% (95%CI 0–70).

Direct mutation analysis of the entire coding region of *BRCA1* and 2 in 38 prostate cancer clusters from the UK Familial Prostate Cancer Study has not revealed any *BRCA1* mutations, although two novel deleterious germline mutations have been found in *BRCA2* (Edwards *et al.* 1998).

Overall, germline mutations in *BRCA1* and *BRCA2* appear to play a limited role in familial prostate cancer. Families with both prostate and breast cancer cases may result from mutations in other predisposition genes.

Low-penetrance genes

In addition to high-penetrance major susceptibility genes, other more common genes with lower penetrance are thought to play a significant role in the inherited predisposition to prostate cancer. The presence of these genes would explain why only limited numbers of families with large numbers of cases exist. Candidate low-penetrance genes are those involved in cellular proliferation and house-keeping activities of the cell.

Prostate cancer is an androgen-dependent tumour. Mutations and/or polymorphisms in any of the genes involved in the androgen pathway could therefore play a role in the development of prostate cancer. Examples include the androgen receptor gene and 5α-reductase gene which converts testosterone to its more active metabolite, dihydrotestosterone.

Androgen receptor

Although the androgen receptor gene has been excluded as a site for a high-penetrance prostate cancer susceptibility gene, it is a candidate for a lower-penetrance gene.

Dihydrotestosterone binds to the androgen receptor forming a complex which is capable of transactivating target genes, thus allowing cellular proliferation. This activity is in the *N*-terminal domain of the androgen receptor which contains expressed trinucleotide repeats. Several studies (Irvine *et al.* 1995; Hardy *et al.* 1996; Giovannucci *et al.* 1997) have shown that there is an association between shorter repeats and prostate cancer risk, and that a smaller repeat is associated with a higher level of receptor transactivation function (Coetzee & Ross 1994). A study of CAG and GGN expressed polymorphic repeats in the androgen receptor gene in 178 systematic prostate cancer cases, compared with geographically matched controls, has not shown any statistically significant association with prostate cancer risk. However, longer GGN repeat length was associated with a halving of disease-free survival on univariate analysis (Edwards *et al.* 1999).

5α-Reductase

Differences in serum testosterone levels and 5α-reductase activity have been proposed as possible explanations for the ethnic differences in prostate cancer incidence. Indeed, among African–Americans where prostate cancer has the highest prevalence, 10–15% higher circulating testosterone levels have been found compared with white individuals (Ross *et al.* 1986). Japanese men who have a very low incidence of the disease have been found to have low levels of 5α-reductase activity (Ross *et al.* 1992). Different allele frequencies for the TA repeat sequence in the 3'-untranslated region of the 5α-reductase gene have been described among African–Americans, whites and Asians (Reichardt *et al.* 1995). Between populations, the length of the TA repeat correlated with risk of prostate cancer but not within populations. Recently, a mis-sense substitution (A49T) in the steroid 5α-reductase gene was found to be associated with an increased incidence of prostate cancer in African– and Hispanic–Americans (Makridakis *et al.* 1999).

We have also studied the 5α-reductase type II gene (*SRD5A2*) for linkage because it is a candidate for a prostate cancer susceptibility gene as a result of its involvement in androgen metabolism. The locus did not show significant evidence of linkage with a point estimate of 25%.

Vitamin D receptor

Men with higher vitamin D_3 levels are at decreased risk of prostate cancer (Boyle 1995). The vitamin D receptor (VDR) has been found to mediate the anti-proliferative effects of vitamin D, and so VDR is another candidate cancer susceptibility gene (Hedlund *et al.* 1996). Ingles *et al.* (1997) genotyped the poly-Amicrosatellite found in VDR and found that men with at least one long (A18–A22) VDR poly(A) allele versus two short (A14–A17) ones had odds ratios of 4.61 (95%CI 1.34–15.82) for developing prostate cancer.

Glutathione-*S*-transferase enzymes

A number of genes involved in the handling of drugs and carcinogens show polymorphic variation. The glutathione-*S*-transferase (GST) gene family is an example. The *GSTM1*, *GSTP1* and *GSTT1* genes that belong to this group code for enzymes involved in phase II metabolism and the elimination of products of oxidative stress. There are well-recognised polymorphisms within these genes which have been associated with an increased susceptibility to various cancers such as bladder, lung and colorectal tumours.

A recent case–control study of 273 early onset prostate cancer cases (diagnosed at age 55 years or younger) found a significant association between the valine/valine genotype at codon 105 in the *GSTP1* gene and prostate cancer risk (= OR; 1.85; 95%CI 1.04–3.06, $p = 0.04$), when compared with the isoleucine/valine or isoleucine/isoleucine genotype at this position (Kote-Jarai *et al.* 2001).

Selenium has been reported to protect against the development of prostate cancer. Thus data are currently being analysed to assess if there is an association between prostate cancer risk and genotypes of the selenium-dependent glutathione enzyme GPX.

Allele loss studies and tumour-suppressor genes

Allele loss or loss of heterozygosity (LOH) tissue studies indicate the sites of tumour-suppressor genes, because in the tumour the wild-type allele is lost. This results in inactivation of the tumour-suppressor gene. Individuals heterozygous for markers in the area of loss therefore have their heterozygous state reduced to a homozygosity, hence the term LOH. The most favoured candidates for sites of tumour-suppressor genes in prostate cancer are chromosomes 8p (Bova *et al.* 1993), 10q, 16q, (Carter *et al.* 1990), 13q (Yin *et al.* 1999) and 18q (Latil *et al.* 1994), because the highest rates of loss have been observed in these regions. In one study of 52 sporadic prostate cancers, loss of 8p was present in 63% of tumours and, in a metastasis, a homozygous deletion at 8p22 has been found. This deletion narrows the area of loss to a 14-cM interval and is strongly suggestive of a tumour-suppressor gene in this region. In 23 tumours from patients with localised prostate cancer, 52% had LOH at 17q and 44% had LOH with a marker within the *BRCA1* gene (Gao *et al.* 1995). A metastasis-suppressor gene at 11p11.2, *KAI1*, has been found by Kawana *et al.* (1997) to play a role in advanced prostate cancer.

Mutations of *TP53* are the most common genetic changes in many cancer types (Hollstein *et al.* 1991). However, in prostate cancer, *TP53* mutation is not very common in primary tumours. Mutations of *TP53* were seen in 25% of 92 tumours in one study by Navone *et al.* (1993), but all the mutations were observed in metastatic tissue and were a late event. Similar results have been obtained for the retinoblastoma gene (Bookstein *et al.* 1990) and the DNA polymerase β gene (Dobashi *et al.* 1994), where changes are more common in metastatic disease than in earlier disease.

Recent LOH studies in a series of 101 tumours, collected through the CRC BPG/UK FPC Study from patients with early onset disease or positive family history, have revealed high rates of loss on chromosomes 1p (35%), 12p (30%) and at *BRCA2* (48%).

Although these are preliminary results and need further confirmation, the locus at 12p is of particular interest because two genomic screens published recently found evidence for linkage to 12p in prostate cancer families (Landis *et al.* 1999; Suarez *et al.* 2000a).

Conclusions

Linkage reports to date have produced mixed results, with no convincing evidence for the role of any one particular locus in the predisposition to prostate cancer.

The greatest linkage evidence is for the 1q24-35 gene.There may be several reasons why this gene has not yet been cloned: the original region of interest was very large (50 cM) compared with other loci identified by linkage such as *BRCA2* (only 3 cM), and so a larger region has to be sequenced in families to discover the candidate code. There have been discrepancies about the exact peak position of linkage from different groups; many suggest it is distal to the original peak reported, and it is not clear whether the 1q42 locus is a separate locus to the 1q24 gene locus.

Other factors may contribute to the problem of confirming linkage: population and ethnic differences between the sample sets are inevitable and undoubtedly complicate the mapping process. Prostate cancer is a common disease and low LOD scores may occur due to the presence of phenocopies, i.e. men who have developed disease that is sporadic and not caused by an inherited germline mutation. Prostate cancer typically occurs at a late age, so it is often difficult to have DNA available from living affected men for more than one generation. The lack of distinguishing features between the hereditary and sporadic forms of the disease is another problem. No significant differences have been found overall between the two groups in terms of clinical stage, pathological stage, Gleason score, tumour volume or preoperative prostate-specific antigen (PSA) value (Valeri *et al.* 2000). Furthermore, various groups have collected families using different case clustering criteria and mode of presentation. It is possible that PSA-detected prostate cancer may, in some instances, behave differently from clinically presenting disease.

Finally, and perhaps most importantly, genetic heterogeneity is a feature of this disease: in other words multiple prostate cancer susceptibility genes are thought to exist. Thus, any one prostate cancer susceptibility locus may be responsible for only a small proportion of families affected by hereditary prostate cancer in general. In the presence of such genetic heterogeneity, it may be difficult for different groups to replicate linkage to an infrequent locus that may account for only a small proportion of families. Evaluation of extended pedigrees with stratified analysis of family subsets and meta-analyses of large datasets are therefore crucial in the successful confirmation of prostate cancer susceptibility loci. Ultimately the only definite evidence will come from direct mutation analysis. This has tremendous implications for the direction of genetic predisposition research in prostate cancer over the next 5 years. An extensive candidate gene approach, even for higher-risk genes may soon be necessary if the proportion of families resulting from each gene is low. For low-penetrance genes, an association study approach is needed but this will require large DNA sample banks and well-characterised clinical data. Advances in robotic technology will greatly help this process.

Acknowledgements

We are most grateful to the Prostate Cancer Charitable Trust which has generously supported prostate cancer research at the Institute of Cancer Research, UK and funded very stimulating meetings, which have resulted in good collaboration worldwide in this field. Funding for our data presented in this review is provided by the Prostate Cancer Charitable Trust, Cancer Research Campaign, the Institute of Cancer Research (UK) and the EU. The genotyping and PCR machines were supported by the Times Christmas Appeal and the Prostate Cancer Charity. The contribution of all the members of the families in the study is gratefully acknowledged. DPD is supported by the Bob Champion Cancer Trust, UK. We would like to thank the Department of Epidemiology, MD Anderson Cancer Center, which initiated the study of familial prostate cancer in Texas.

References

Ahman AK, Jonsson BA, Damber JE, BerghA, Emanuelsson M, Gronberg H (2000). Low frequency of allelic imbalance at the prostate cancer susceptibility loci HPC1 and 1p36 in Swedish men with hereditary prostate cancer. *Genes Chromosomes and Cancer* **29**, 292–296

Anderson DE & Badzioch MD (1992). Breast cancer risks in relatives of male breast cancer patients. *Journal of the National Cancer Institute* **84**, 1114–1117

Badzioch M, Eeles R, Le Blanc G (2000). Suggestive evidence for a site specific prostate cancer gene on chromosome 1p36. The Cer/BPG UK Familial Prostate Cancer Study Co-ordinators and Collaborators. The EU Biomed Collaborators. *Journal of Medical Genetics* **37**, 947–949

Bergerheim US, Kunimi K, Collins VP, Ekman P (1991). Deletion mapping of chromosomes 8, 10, and 16 in human prostatic carcinoma. *Genes Chromosomes and Cancer* **3**, 215–220

Bergthorsson J, Johannesdottir G, Arason A *et al.* (2000). Analysis of HPC1, HPCX, and PCaP in Icelandic hereditary prostate cancer. *Human Genetics* **107**, 372–375

Berry R, Schaid DJ, Smith JR *et al.* (2000a). Linkage analyses at the chromosome 1 loci 1q24-25 (HPC1), 1q42.2-43 (PCAP), and 1p36 (CAPB) in families with hereditary prostate cancer. *American Journal of Human Genetics* **66**, 539–546

Berry R, Schroeder JJ, French AJ *et al.* (2000b). Evidence for a prostate cancer-susceptibility locus on chromosome 20. *American Journal of Human Genetics* **67**, 82–91

Berthon P, Valeri A, Cohen-Akenine A *et al.* (1998). Predisposing gene for early-onset prostate cancer, localized on chromosome 1q42.2-43. *American Journal of Human Genetics* **62**, 1416–1424

Bookstein R, Rio P, Madreperla SA *et al.* (1990). Promoter deletion and loss of retinoblastoma gene expression in human prostate carcinoma. *Proceedings of the National Academy of Science USA* **87**, 7762–7766

Bova GS, Carter BS, Bussemakers MJ *et al.* (1993). Homozygous deletion and frequent allelic loss of chromosome 8p22 loci in human prostate cancer. *Cancer Research* **53**, 3869–3873

Boyle P (1995). Aetiology of prostate cancer. In Garraway M (ed.) *Epidemiology of Prostate Disease*. Edinburgh: Churchill Livingstone, pp 202–213

Breast Cancer Linkage Consortium (1999). Cancer risks in *BRCA2* mutation carriers. *Journal of the National Cancer Institute* **91**, 1310–1316

Cannon LA (1982). Genetic epidemiology of prostate cancer in the Utah Mormon Genealogy. *Cancer Surveys* **1**, 47–69

Cannon-Albright LA, Goldgar DE, Meyer LJ *et al.* (1992). Assignment of a locus for familial melanoma, MLM, to chromosome 9p13- p22 [see comments]. *Science* **258**, 1148–1152

Carter BS, Ewing CM, Ward WS *et al.* WB (1990). Allelic loss of chromosomes 16q and 10q in human prostate cancer. *Proceedings of the National Academy of Science of the USA* **87**, 8751–8755

Carter BS, Beaty TH, Steinberg GD, Childs B, Walsh PC (1992). Mendelian inheritance of familial prostate cancer. *Proceedings of the National Academy of Science of the USA* **89**, 3367–3371

Coetzee GA & Ross RK (1994). Re: Prostate cancer and the androgen receptor [letter]. *Journal of the National Cancer Institute* **86**, 872–873

Coleman MP *et al.* (1993). *Trends in Cancer Incidence and Mortality*. Lyon: IARC

Cooney KA, McCarthy JD, Lange E *et al.* (1997). Prostate cancer susceptibility locus on chromosome 1q: a confirmatory study [see comments]. *Journal of the National Cancer Institute* **89**, 955–959

Dijkman GA & Debruyne FM (1996). Epidemiology of prostate cancer. *European Urology* **30**, 281–295

Dobashi Y, Shuin T, Tsuruga H, Uemura H, Torigoe S, Kubota Y (1994). DNA polymerase beta gene mutation in human prostate cancer. *Cancer Research* **54**, 2827–2829

Dunsmuir WD, Edwards SM, Lakhani SR *et al.* (1998). Allelic imbalance in familial and sporadic prostate cancer at the putative human prostate cancer susceptibility locus, HPC1. CRC/BPG UK Familial Prostate Cancer Study Collaborators. Cancer Research Campaign/British Prostate Group. *British Journal of Cancer* **78**, 1430–1433

Edwards SM, Dunsmuir WD, Gillett CE *et al.* (1998). Immunohistochemical expression of BRCA2 protein and allelic loss at the BRCA2 locus in prostate cancer. CRC/BPG UK Familial Prostate Cancer Study Collaborators. *International Journal of Cancer* **78**, 1–7

Edwards SM, Badzioch MD, Minter R *et al.* (1999). Androgen receptor polymorphisms: association with prostate cancer risk, relapse and overall survival. *International Journal of Cancer* **84**, 458–465

Eeles RA, Durocher F, Edwards S *et al.* (1998). Linkage analysis of chromosome 1q markers in 136 prostate cancer families. The Cancer Research Campaign/British Prostate Group UK. Familial Prostate Cancer Study Collaborators. *American Journal of Human Genetics* **62**, 653–658

Eeles RA, the UK Familial Prostate Study Co-ordinating Group and the CRC/BPG UK Familial Prostate Cancer Study Collaborators (1999). Genetic predisposition to prostate cancer. In *Prostate Cancer and Prostatic Diseases* **2**, 9–15

Ford D, Easton DF, Bishop DT, Narod SA, Goldgar DE (1994). Risks of cancer in BRCA1-mutation carriers. Breast Cancer Linkage Consortium. *The Lancet* **343**, 692–695

Gao X, Zacharek A, Salkowski A *et al.* (1995). Loss of heterozygosity of the BRCA1 and other loci on chromosome 17q in human prostate cancer. *Cancer Research* **55**, 1002–1005

Gibbs M, Chakrabarti L, Stanford JL *et al.* (1999a). Analysis of chromosome 1q42.2-43 in 152 families with high risk of prostate cancer. *American Journal of Human Genetics* **64**, 1087–1095

Gibbs M, Stanford JL, McIndoe RA *et al.* (1999b). Evidence for a rare prostate cancer-susceptibility locus at chromosome 1p36. *American Journal of Human Genetics* **64**, 776–787

Gibbs M, Stanford JL, Jarvik GP *et al.* (2000). A genomic scan of families with prostate cancer identifies multiple regions of interest. *American Journal of Human Genetics* **67**,100–109

Giovannucci E, Stampfer MJ, Krithivas K *et al.* (1997). The CAG repeat within the androgen receptor gene and its relationship to prostate cancer [published erratum appears in *Proc Natl Acad Sci USA* 1997; **94**: 8272]. *Proceedings of the National Academy of Science of the USA* **94**, 3320–3323

Goldgar DE, Easton DF, Cannon-Albright LA, Skolnick MH (1994). Systematic population-based assessment of cancer risk in first-degree relatives of cancer probands. *Journal of the National Cancer Institute* **86**, 1600–1608

Goode EL, Stanford JL, Chakrabarti L *et al.* (2000a). Linkage analysis of 150 high-risk prostate cancer families at 1q24-25. *Genetics and Epidemiology* **18**, 251–275

Goode EL, Stanford JL, Gibbs M *et al.* (2000b). Incorporating clinical data into analysis of susceptibility loci suggests CAPB linkage among prostate cancer families with a high-grade case. *American Journal of Human Genetics* **67**(4, Suppl 2), 329

Grönberg H, Damber L, Damber JE (1994). Studies of genetic factors in prostate cancer in a twin population. *Journal of Urology* **152**, 1484–1487

Grönberg H, Damber L, Damber JE, Iselius L (1997a). Segregation analysis of prostate cancer in Sweden: support for dominant inheritance. *American Journal of Epidemiology* **146**, 552–557

Grönberg H, Isaacs SD, Smith JR *et al.* (1997b). Characteristics of prostate cancer in families potentially linked to the hereditary prostate cancer 1 (HPC1) locus [see comments]. *Journal of the American Medical Association* **278**, 1251–1255

Hall JM, Lee MK, Newman B *et al.* (1990). Linkage of early-onset familial breast cancer to chromosome 17q21. *Science* **250**, 1684–1689

Hardy DO, Scher HI, Bogenreider T *et al.* (1996). Androgen receptor CAG repeat lengths in prostate cancer: correlation with age of onset. *Journal of Clinical Endocrinology and Metabolism* **81**, 4400–4405

Hedlund TE, Moffatt KA, Miller GJ (1996). Vitamin D receptor expression is required for growth modulation by 1 alpha,25-dihydroxyvitamin D3 in the human prostatic carcinoma cell line ALVA-31. *Journal of Steroid Biochemistry and Molecular Biology* **58**, 277–288

Hollstein M, Sidransky D, Vogelstein B, Harris CC (1991). p53 mutations in human cancers. *Science* **253**, 49–53

Hsieh CL, Oakley-Girvan I, Gallagher RP *et al.* (1997). Re: prostate cancer susceptibility locus on chromosome 1q: a confirmatory study [letter; comment]. *Journal of the National Cancer Institute* **89**, 1893–1894

Ingles SA, Ross RK, Yu MC *et al.* (1997). Association of prostate cancer risk with genetic polymorphisms in vitamin D receptor and androgen receptor [see comments]. *Journal of the National Cancer Institute* **89**, 166–170

Irvine RA, Yu MC, Ross RK, Coetzee GA (1995). The CAG and GGC microsatellites of the androgen receptor gene are in linkage disequilibrium in men with prostate cancer. *Cancer Research* **55**, 1937–1940

Kawana Y, Komiya A, Ueda T *et al.* (1997). Location of KAI1 on the short arm of human chromosome 11 and frequency of allelic loss in advanced human prostate cancer. *Prostate* **32**, 205–213

Kote-Jarai Z, Easten D, Edwards SM *et al.* (2001). Relationship between glutathione-*S*-transferase M, P and T, polymorphisms and early onset prostate cancer. *Pharmacogenetics* **11**, 325–330

Landis SH, Murray T, Bolden S, Wingo PA (1999). Cancer statistics, 1999 [see comments]. *CA: A Cancer Journal for Clinicians* **49**, 8–31

Lange EM, Chen H, Brierley K *et al.* (1999). Linkage analysis of 153 prostate cancer families over a 30-cM region containing the putative susceptibility locus HPCX. *Clinical Cancer Research* **5**, 4013–4020

Latil A, Baron JC, Cussenot O *et al.* (1994). Genetic alterations in localized prostate cancer: identification of a common region of deletion on chromosome arm 18q. *Genes Chromosomes and Cancer* **11**, 119–125

McIndoe RA, Stanford JL, Gibbs M *et al.* (1997). Linkage analysis of 49 high-risk families does not support a common familial prostate cancer-susceptibility gene at 1q24-25. *American Journal of Human Genetics* **61**, 347–353

Makridakis NM, Ross RK, Pike MC *et al.* (1999). Association of mis-sense substitution in SRD5A2 gene with prostate cancer in African-American and Hispanic men in Los Angeles, USA. *The Lancet* **354**, 975–978

Morganti G & Aea GLC (1956). Recherches clinico-statistiques et génétiques sur les néoplasies de la prostate. *Acta Genetica Statistica* **6**, 304–305

Navone NM, Troncoso P, Pisters LL *et al.* (1993). p53 protein accumulation and gene mutation in the progression of human prostate carcinoma. *Journal of the National Cancer Institute* **85**, 1657–1669

Neuhausen SL, Farnham JM, Kort E, Tavtigian SV, Skolnick MH, Cannon-Albright LA (1999). Prostate cancer susceptibility locus HPC1 in Utah high-risk pedigrees. *Human Molecular Genetics* **8**, 2437–2442

Office for National Statistics (2000). *Cancer Survival Trends in England and Wales 1971–1995*. No. 61, Series SMP5. London: HMSO

Parkin DM, Pisani P, Ferlay J (1993). Estimates of the worldwide incidence of eighteen major cancers in 1985. *International Journal of Cancer* **54**, 594–606

Reichardt JK, Makridakis N, Henderson BE, Yu MC, Pike MC, Ross RK (1995). Genetic variability of the human SRD5A2 gene: implications for prostate cancer risk. *Cancer Research* **55**, 3973–3975

Ross R, Bernstein L, Judd H, Hanisch R, Pike M, Henderson B (1986). Serum testosterone levels in healthy young black and white men. *Journal of the National Cancer Institute* **76**, 45–48

Ross RK, Bernstein L, Lobo RA *et al.* (1992). 5-alpha-reductase activity and risk of prostate cancer among Japanese and US white and black males. *The Lancet* **339**, 887–889

Schaid DJ, McDonnell SK, Blute ML, Thibodeau SN (1998). Evidence for autosomal dominant inheritance of prostate cancer. *American Journal of Human Genetics* **62**, 1425–1438

Sellers TA, Potter JD, Rich SS *et al.* (1994). Familial clustering of breast and prostate cancers and risk of postmenopausal breast cancer [see comments]. *Journal of the National Cancer Institute* **86**, 1860–1865

Singh R and the ACTANE Consortium (2000). No evidence of linkage to chromosome 1q 42.2– 4.3 in 131 prostate cancer families from the ACTANE Consortium. *British Journal of Cancer* **83**, 1654–1658

Smith JR, Freije D, Carpten JD *et al.* (1996). Major susceptibility locus for prostate cancer on chromosome 1 suggested by a genome-wide search [see comments]. *Science* **274**, 1371–1374

Steinberg GD, Carter BS, Beaty TH, Childs B, Walsh PC (1990). Family history and the risk of prostate cancer. *Prostate* **17**, 337–347

Suarez BK, Lin J, Burmester JK *et al.* (2000a). A genome screen of multiplex sibships with prostate cancer. *American Journal of Human Genetics* **66**, 933–944

Suarez BK, Lin J, Witte JS *et al.* (2000b). Replication linkage study for prostate cancer susceptibility genes [In Process Citation]. *Prostate* **45**, 106–114

Tavtigian SV *et al.* (2000). A strong candidate prostate cancer predisposition gene at chromosome 17p. *American Journal of Human Genetics* **67**, 11

Thiessen EU (1974). Concerning a familial association between breast cancer and both prostatic and uterine malignancies. *Cancer* **34**, 1102–1107

Tulinius H, Egilsson V, Olafsdottir GH, Sigvaldason H (1992). Risk of prostate, ovarian, and endometrial cancer among relatives of women with breast cancer. *British Medical Journal* **305**, 855–857

Valeri A, Azzouzi R, Drelon E *et al.* (2000). Early-onset hereditary prostate cancer is not associated with specific clinical and biological features. *Prostate* **45**, 66–71

Whittemore AS, Lin IG, Oakley-Girvan I *et al.* (1999). No evidence of linkage for chromosome 1q42.2-43 in prostate cancer [letter]. *American Journal of Human Genetics* **65**, 254–256

Whittemore AS, Wu AH, Kolonel LN *et al.* (1995). Family history and prostate cancer risk in black, white, and Asian men in the United States and Canada. *American Journal of Epidemiology* **141**, 732–740

Woolf CM (1960). An investigation of the familial aspects of carcinoma of the prostate. *Cancer* **13**, 739–744

Wooster R, Neuhausen SL, Mangion J *et al.* (1994). Localization of a breast cancer susceptibility gene, BRCA2, to chromosome 13q12-13. *Science* **265**, 2088–2090

Xu J (2000a). Combined analysis of hereditary prostate cancer linkage to 1q24-25: results from 772 hereditary prostate cancer families from the International Consortium for Prostate Cancer Genetics. *American Journal of Human Genetics* **66**, 945–957

Xu J (2000b). Combined analysis of hereditary prostate cancer linkage to 1q24-25: results from 772 hereditary prostate cancer families from the International Consortium for Prostate Cancer Genetics. *American Journal of Human Genetics* **67** (erratum)

Xu J, Meyers D, Freije D *et al.* (1998). Evidence for a prostate cancer susceptibility locus on the X chromosome. *Nature Genetics* **20**, 175–179

Yin Z, Spitz MR, Babaian RJ, Strom SS, Troncoso P, Kagan J (1999). Limiting the location of a putative human prostate cancer tumor suppressor gene at chromosome 13q14.3. *Oncogene* **18**, 7576–7583

Chapter 2

The epidemiology of prostate cancer: rates and risk factor

Naomi E Allen and Timothy J Key

Introduction

Prostate cancer is the second most common cancer among men in the UK, accounting for approximately 20,000 cancer cases and 10,000 deaths each year (Office for National Statistics 2000). With the ageing of the population and the continuing decline in other common cancers, such as those of the lung and stomach (Figure 2.1), prostate cancer is becoming an increasing public health burden. This chapter aims to give a description of the geographical and temporal trends in prostate cancer incidence and mortality, focusing on trends observed in the USA and the UK. An outline of the risk factors involved in the aetiology of the disease is then provided, with an emphasis on the roles of hormonal and dietary factors.

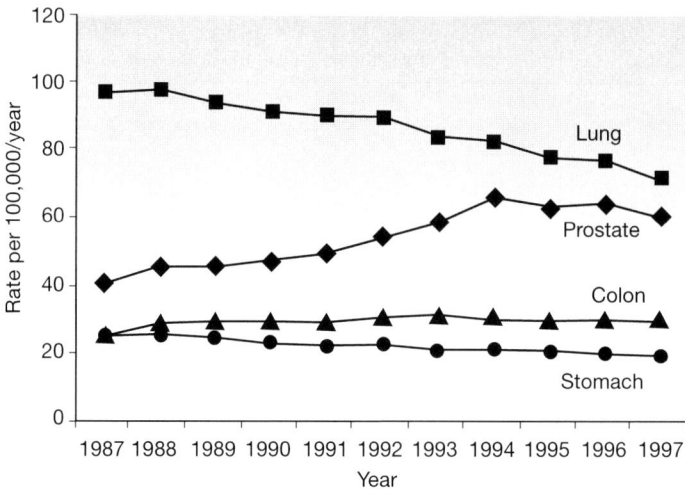

Figure 2.1 Trends in common cancer incidence rates in men, England and Wales, 1987–1997. Rates are age standardised using the European Standard population. Note that the figures for 1995–1997 are provisional only. (From Office for National Statistics 2000.)

Descriptive epidemiology
Clinical and latent disease

Postmortem studies have shown that between 30 and 40% of men aged 50 years and over have small, well-differentiated tumours within the peripheral zone of the prostate gland (Breslow *et al.* 1977). By the age of 80, microscopically detected prostatic adenocarcinoma is present in 70–80% of all men (Akazaki & Stemmerman 1973). The majority of these tumours grow relatively slowly and never manifest themselves clinically, so that most men with microscopic tumours die of other causes. These so-called 'latent' prostate tumours are usually found incidentally at autopsy or during routine surgical procedures, such as transurethral resection for the prostate (TURP), which is commonly used for the treatment of benign prostatic hyperplasia. TURP procedures are routinely followed by histological evaluation of the tissue removed from the periurethral area and, in as many as 15% of cases, this reveals small and previously unsuspected malignancies (Rohr 1987). Measurements of prostate-specific antigen (PSA), a protease enzyme produced by prostatic epithelial cells and whose serum concentration is increased in malignancy, have also allowed much earlier detection of asymptomatic prostate cancer (Crawford & DeAntoni 1993). Indeed, PSA testing is used for the purpose of monitoring disease status in patients and, in countries such as the USA (Chodak 1994) and Australia (Ward *et al.* 1998), is widely used for aiding the detection of prostate cancer, although there is, as yet, no systematic screening for prostate cancer in these countries.

The extent to which these medical procedures lead to the early diagnosis of tumours that would eventually cause symptoms, or to the detection of latent disease that would never become symptomatic, is not clear. The *International Classification of Diseases* does not distinguish between tumours found incidentally and those associated with clinical symptoms, so the impact of such procedures on the rates of prostate cancer being detected and subsequently registered as incident cancer may be substantial.

Geographical trends in prostate cancer incidence and mortality
Incidence

There is a 30-fold variation in prostate cancer incidence rates reported between populations. The highest reported rates of incident prostate cancer are found in the USA (>100/100,000 per year); intermediate rates are found in western Europe (around 30–50/100,000 per year), and the lowest rates are seen in Asian countries (<10/100,000 per year) (IARC 1997) (Figure 2.2). In the USA, prostate cancer accounts for approximately 32% of all male incident cancers; in the UK it accounts for about 15% of all cancers in men, and in China less than 1% of all incident cancers in men.

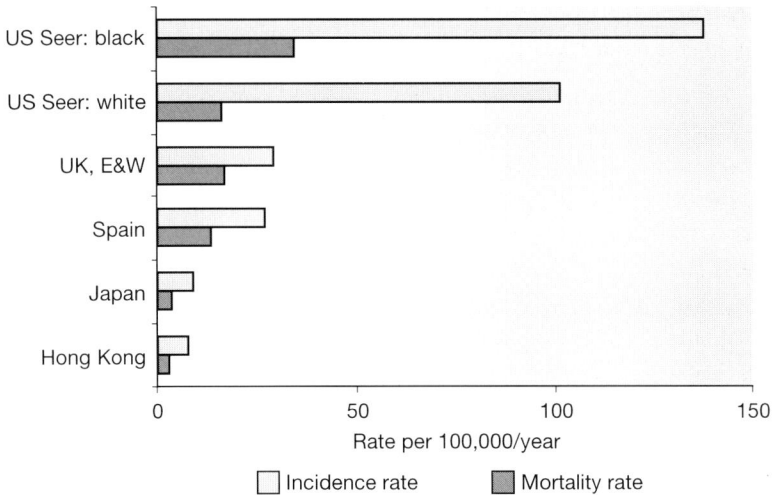

Figure 2.2 Prostate cancer incidence and mortality rates, 1992–1998, in selected countries. Rates are age standardised to the World Standard population. Incidence rates are derived from IARC (1997); mortality rates are derived from the WHO Cancer Mortality database (1998).

A substantial part of the variation in reported incidence rates can be attributed to differences in medical practices between countries, such as the use of TURP procedures and PSA testing. Indeed, it has been estimated that the current low incidence rate in Japan would increase by three- to fourfold after taking American-based methods of detection, diagnosis and cancer registration into consideration (Shimizu *et al.* 1991). Despite such corrections, however, incidence rates in Japan would still remain approximately 50% lower than those found in men of Japanese ancestry in the USA and up to 75% lower than white American men.

Mortality

Although the large variation in prostate cancer incidence rates may result partly from differences in detection of latent disease, there also exists a three- to fourfold variation in mortality rates between high- and low-risk countries (Figure 2.2). Despite the much higher incidence rates among white men in the USA compared with the UK, age-adjusted mortality rates in these two countries are similar at about 15/100,000 deaths per year. In contrast, mortality rates in Japan are much lower at approximately 5/100,000 deaths per year (World Health Organization 1998). This suggests that differences in detection cannot explain all of the disparities in incidence rates between countries and that there are real differences between populations in the rates of development of prostate cancer to a clinical and ultimately fatal form.

Secular trends in prostate cancer incidence and mortality

Incidence

The rates of incident prostate cancers have increased dramatically in recent years in both low- and high-incidence countries, by an average of 3% annually worldwide (IARC 1997). The annual number of new cases of prostate cancer registered in the UK increased by 79% between 1987 and 1994, from 10,837 to 19,399 and thereafter fell slightly to 18,300 cases in 1997. Age-standardised incidence rates increased by approximately 3% per year during the 1980s and increased more rapidly in the early 1990s, with an overall increase of 61% from 41 to 66/100,000 between 1987 and 1994 (see Figure 2.1), with a slight fall thereafter to 61/100,000 in 1997. The increase observed throughout the late 1980s and early 1990s occurred across all age groups, although it was most apparent in the 55 to 64-year age group, increasing by 168% between 1987 and 1996 alone (Figure 2.3).

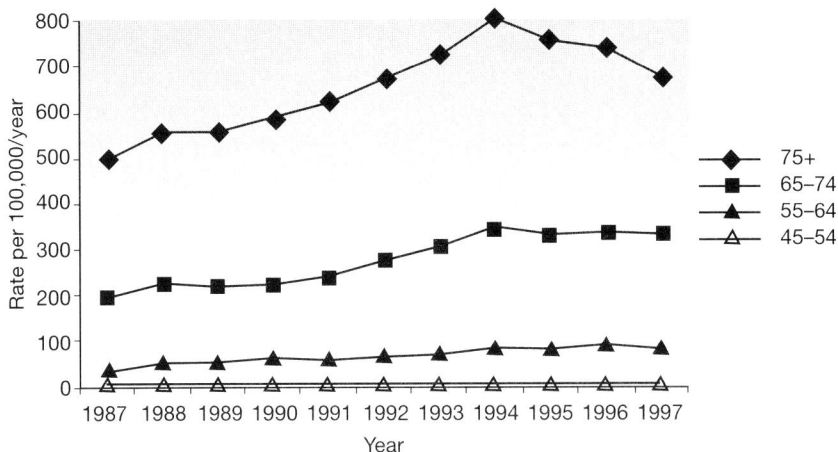

Figure 2.3 Age-specific trends in prostate cancer incidence, England and Wales, 1987–1997. Data for 1995–1997 are provisional only. (From Office for National Statistics (1984–1994); Office for National Statistics 2000.)

This rapid increase in incidence can be largely explained by the increasing use of TURP procedures in the late 1980s, as seen in the USA (Potosky *et al.* 1990), followed by the gradual introduction of PSA testing in the early 1990s, leading to increased detection of incidental tumours (Brewster *et al.* 2000). Indeed, the use of PSA as a screening tool in many parts of the USA corresponded with a 61% increase in age-adjusted prostate cancer incidence between 1986 and 1992 for white men (Legler *et al.* 1998). It is interesting to note that this 61% increase was associated with a maximum of 19% of white men aged 65 years or older across the USA having had a first PSA test (Legler *et al.* 1998). This implies that, if a higher proportion of men had been given a first PSA test, the incidence might have increased several-fold.

The incidence rate is now showing evidence of a decline in the USA by approximately 10% per year, which began in 1992 (Oliver *et al.* 2000). As discussed above, provisional data for the UK also suggest that prostate cancer incidence rates have started to decline since 1995 (see Figure 2.1) (Office for National Statistics 2000). This has been attributed to the removal of prevalent cases from the population by previous PSA testing and a decreased use of TURP procedures in both countries (Chamberlain *et al.* 1997; Merrill *et al.* 1999).

Changes in medical procedures may therefore largely explain the observed trends in incident cancer over time. However, it is still possible that a small proportion of the increase observed during the late 1980s and early 1990s may have been genuine and caused by increased exposure to some, as yet unidentified, risk factor(s).

Mortality

In contrast to incidence data, prostate cancer mortality rates have remained relatively stable over the last 10 years in the UK, contrasting with mortality rates for cancers of the lung and stomach, which have declined by 26% and 33%, respectively (Figure 2.4). Although overall mortality data are not affected by artefacts such as increased detection and ascertainment, they must be interpreted with some caution if used as indicators of the incidence of aggressive prostate cancer. This is because changes in assigning causes of death and, perhaps, improved treatment can explain some of the observed trends with time. Indeed, the slight increase in mortality rates in the UK between 1986 and 1992 (Figure 2.4) was most likely the result of a change in the rules for coding the underlying cause of death in England and Wales (Grulich *et al.* 1995). This lead to a reduction in deaths coded as caused by terminal events and an increase in deaths coded as resulting from underlying causes such as cancer. This change had the greatest impact among elderly men and the prostate cancer mortality rate in men over the age of 85 years increased by approximately 23% in the late 1980s and early 1990s (Figure 2.5).

Similarly, the small increase observed in the USA in the late 1980s (Figure 2.6) may have been the result of artefact in that more men may have had their death ascribed to the disease because they had previously been diagnosed with prostate cancer (Feuer *et al.* 1999). The mortality rate is now showing evidence of a decline, by approximately 3.8% per year in the USA, and by 1.7% per year in the UK, which began in 1991 and 1995 respectively (Figure 2.6). There has been some speculation that PSA testing and early treatment of localised disease may be partly responsible for this recent trend (Etzioni *et al.* 1999), but the overall low prevalence of PSA testing and the early date at which mortality started to decline make this unlikely. It is more probable that improvement in overall management, treatment and subsequent survival of men with prostate cancer has caused the recent fall in the mortality rate. Randomised controlled trials are now under way to establish whether PSA screening reduces mortality rates (Gohagan *et al.* 1994; Moon *et al.* 1995; Schroeder *et al.* 1996), and results from these studies will be available in the next few years.

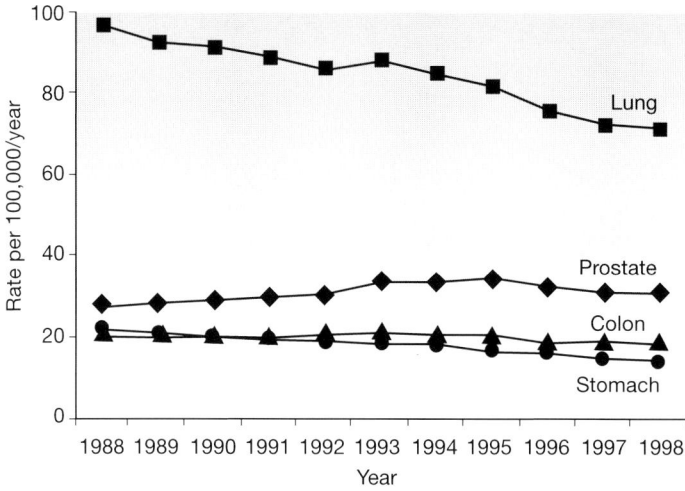

Figure 2.4 Trends in common cancer mortality rates in men, England and Wales, 1988–1998. Rates are age standardised using England and Wales Standard population. (From Office for National Statistics 1988–1998.)

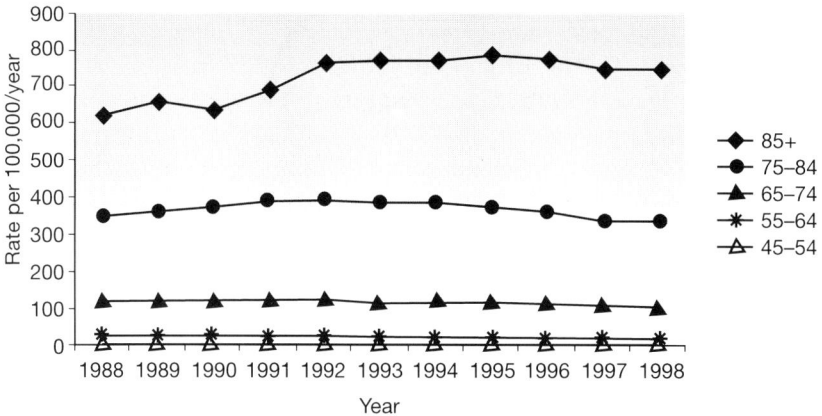

Figure 2.5 Trends in prostate cancer mortality by age, England and Wales, 1988–1998. Rates are age standardised using England and Wales Standard population. (From Office for National Statistics 1988–1998.)

In contrast to Western countries, prostate cancer mortality in low-risk countries has increased. In Japan, for example, mortality rates have increased by approximately 50% from 3.5 to 5.2/100,000 per year between 1986 and 1996 (Figure 2.6). Such an increase strongly suggests that changes in exposure to environmental risk factors, such as the increasing adoption of a Western lifestyle and corresponding changes in

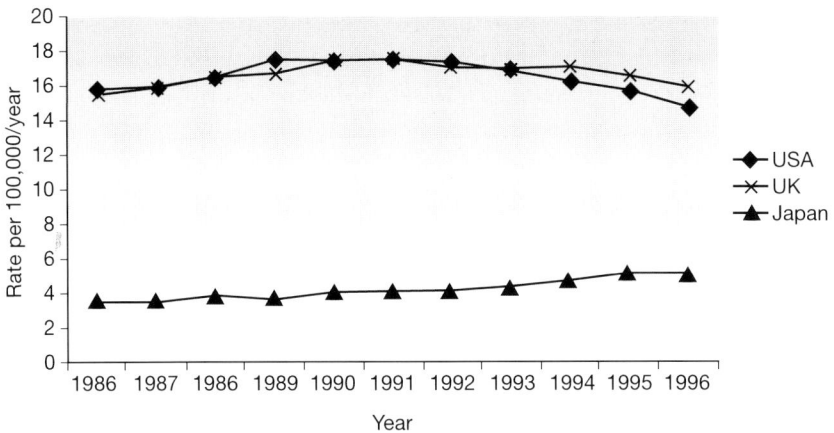

Figure 2.6 Prostate cancer mortality in the USA, the UK and Japan, 1986–1996. Rates are age standardised to the World Standard population. (From WHO Cancer Mortality database 1998.)

dietary habits may influence the progression of prostate cancer to a clinical and fatal form.

Risk factors

No risk factors have been established for prostate cancer other than age, ethnicity and a family history of the disease. Descriptive epidemiological data suggest that endogenous hormones and/or environmental exposures, such as diet, may play an important role in prostate carcinogenesis. Evidence that factors such as obesity, tobacco smoking, alcohol consumption, occupational exposures, diabetes, sexual activity and sexually transmitted diseases, vasectomy and physical activity are related to prostate cancer is inconsistent and has been reviewed elsewhere (Nomura & Kolonel 1991; Mettlin 1997).

Age

Prostate cancer incidence and mortality increase significantly with increasing age – more so than for any other cancer, starting later in life (especially over the age of 70 years) and then rising sharply with increasing age (Cook *et al.* 1969). In the UK, men over the age of 85 years have a 70-fold increased risk of developing clinical prostate cancer compared with men aged 50–54 years, with an incidence rate of 1,052/ 100,000 and a mortality of 750/100,000 per year (see Figure 2.3).

Ethnicity

As previously mentioned, there is a large variation in prostate cancer incidence rates reported between populations, with the incidence being highest among African–Americans, intermediate among European white men and lowest among Asian men (IARC 1997) (see Figure 2.2). However, little is known about why African–American men have a higher incidence compared with white men in the USA. The differences in incidence could, in theory, be due to differences in screening availability and detection of the disease, but this seems unlikely because, if anything, African–American men would be expected to receive less medical investigation than white men. Further, there are even larger differences in mortality between these ethnic groups, with African–Americans having approximately 120% higher mortality rates than white men (see Figure 2.2). This strongly suggests that environmental and/or genetic factors, which differ between ethnic groups within the USA, may affect the progression of disease from a latent to a clinical form.

Data on prostate cancer rates in African men are sparse, being based on a few regional registries, the reported age-standardised incidence rates of which vary from 2.3/100,000 in Setif, Algeria to 29/100,000 in Harare, Zimbabwe (IARC 1997). However, detection and registration of prostate cancer may be underestimated in African countries and prospective data from a small hospital series suggests that African men in Nigeria may actually have a similar high risk to that of African–American men (Osegbe 1997). If this is substantiated, it would further strengthen the role for genetic factors in explaining differences in prostate cancer between ethnic groups.

The fact that the low rates of prostate cancer in Japan are increasing and that men who migrate from Japan to the USA have an increased risk of developing the disease supports a strong role for environmental factors in prostate cancer progression. Indeed, migrant studies have shown that Japanese immigrants to the USA have at least a fourfold increase in prostate cancer mortality rates (Haenzel & Hurihara 1968). These findings therefore suggest that migration and exposure to different environmental risk factors such as diet may affect prostate cancer risk. However, the observation that incidence and mortality rates among Asian migrants remain lower than those of white Americans and much lower than those of African–Americans implies that genetic factors are also likely to be important determinants of prostate cancer risk.

Family history

The previous chapter in this volume discusses the influence of genetic factors in relation to prostate cancer development and this topic is not reviewed in detail here. However, it should be noted that a family history of prostate cancer is a strong risk factor for this disease. Clinical and epidemiological studies of familial risk of prostate cancer show a trend of increasing risk with increasing number of affected relatives and an earlier age of onset in affected relatives (Carter *et al.* 1990). Evidence suggests that one or more autosomal dominant genes may lead to early onset prostate cancer (Carter *et al.* 1993), although to date the gene(s) in question has not been identified. Although it has been estimated that such gene(s) account for only a small proportion of prostate cancer in the general population, a study of twins in northern Europe indicated that heritable factors might explain as much as 40% of prostate cancer risk (Lichtenstein *et al.* 2000). Genetic factors that carry a moderate effect and are not manifested in a family history may therefore play a significant role in prostate cancer development. Of most interest are polymorphisms found in genes that encode for enzymes involved in androgen metabolism and genes that encode for hormone receptors. Several polymorphisms in these genes have been found to differ between prostate cancer cases and controls (Giovannucci *et al.* 1997; Ingles *et al.* 1997b; Febbo *et al.* 1999; Lunn *et al.* 1999) and to differ in frequency between ethnic groups considered being differentially 'at risk' for prostate cancer (Reichardt *et al.* 1995; Devgan *et al.* 1997; Ingles *et al.* 1997a; Makridakis *et al.* 1999). These relationships should be clarified over the next few years.

Hormones

The steroid sex hormones, androgens and oestrogens, are mitogens that stimulate cell growth; they are necessary for the normal growth and development of the prostate gland. Following the observation that prolonged administration of high levels of testosterone can induce prostate adenocarcinoma in several rat strains (Noble 1977), a causal relationship between sex hormones and prostate cancer has been considered biologically plausible. Testosterone within prostatic cells is converted by 5α-reductase to the more potent dihydrotestosterone (DHT), which is the principal growth-regulating androgen. However, the serum concentration of DHT has limited value as a marker of intraprostatic androgen metabolism because much of it is derived from the skin. Most DHT in the prostate is metabolised to androstanediol (A-diol), which is conjugated to its glucuronide form (A-diol-g) in the liver before excretion (Rittmaster *et al.* 1993). The serum concentration of A-diol-g is thought to be a reasonably specific marker of 5α-reductase activity and intraprostatic DHT (Rittmaster *et al.* 1993).

A meta-analysis of eight published prospective studies has shown that circulating levels of total testosterone do not appear to be related to prostate cancer development (Eaton *et al.* 1999). Serum bioavailable testosterone levels were also similar between men who subsequently developed prostate cancer compared with healthy individuals, although the pooled estimate for bioavailable testosterone is based on too few cases for reliable interpretation. Serum levels of A-diol-g were found to be 5% higher (95% confidence interval, 0–11) in 644 prostate cancer cases compared with 1,048 healthy individuals (Eaton *et al.* 1999). Such differences in serum levels of A-diol-g may reflect larger differences in DHT itself within the prostate gland, leading to an increase in prostate cancer risk.

Circulating levels of insulin-like growth factor-I (IGF-I), a polypeptide hormone that directly stimulates growth of both normal (Culig *et al.* 1996) and cancerous cells within the prostate gland (Connolly & Rose 1994), have also been shown to be higher in men who subsequently go on to develop prostate cancer compared with healthy individuals (Chan *et al.* 1998b; Harman *et al.* 2000; Stattin *et al.* 2000). Environmental or genetic factors that affect sex hormone and/or growth factor metabolism may therefore have important implications in the development of this disease from a latent to a clinical form.

Diet

The evidence from migrant studies suggests that environmental factors play an important role in the development of clinical prostate cancer. Ecological studies suggest that this could be due to the adoption of a Western lifestyle and, in particular, a Western-style diet characterised by energy-rich foods high in refined carbohydrate, meat and dairy products, with a low proportion of energy derived from cereals and other starchy foods (Armstrong & Doll 1975; Rose *et al.* 1986).

Although the data from prospective studies have not established definite causal or protective associations for specific nutrients or dietary factors (World Cancer Research Fund 1997), several hypotheses have emerged. Many early epidemiological studies implicated dietary fat, especially saturated or animal fat, as a risk factor for prostate cancer, although the evidence from later studies has not supported this hypothesis (Kolonel *et al.* 1999). Dairy products and animal protein have also been associated with increased risk (Chan *et al.* 1998a) but the data are inconsistent. Antioxidants have been purported to be protective against prostate cancer, although there is now strong evidence from three large randomised trials that β-carotene, an antioxidant carotenoid, has no beneficial effect (Hennekens *et al.* 1996; Omenn *et al.* 1996; Heinonen *et al.* 1998). Vitamin E supplementation was found to be associated with a significant reduction in prostate cancer rates in a randomised controlled trial in Finland (Heinonen *et al.* 1998), although observational studies have shown mixed results (Chan *et al.* 1999; Eichholzer *et al.* 1999; Gann *et al.* 1999). There is some evidence that other antioxidants such as lycopene (Giovannucci *et al.* 1995; Gann *et al.* 1999) and selenium (Clark *et al.* 1996; Yoshizawa *et al.* 1998) have a protective effect on prostate cancer, although the data are inconsistent (Thomas 1999; Kristal & Cohen 2000).

Ecological comparisons have shown prostate cancer to be much rarer in Asian populations where soya-bean consumption is high, in comparison with Western countries where soya-bean consumption is relatively low. It has been suggested that isoflavones predominantly found in soya-beans might have a protective effect (Messina *et al.* 1994), but the data from analytical studies are sparse and the results inconsistent (Moyad 1999).

If diet is of aetiological importance in prostate cancer development, a possible explanation of its action could be through its effect on hormone metabolism. However, diet does not appear to affect circulating levels of bioavailable androgens, which have been found to be similar in men from different dietary groups (Allen *et al.* 2000). This suggests that dietary differences may not be sufficient to alter the homoeostatic control of bioavailable testosterone (Allen & Key 2000). Perhaps of more importance is the established effect of diet on circulating IGF-I levels (Thissen *et al.* 1994). A diet low in energy and protein and, in particular, a diet low in essential amino acids, has been found to reduce substantially serum IGF-I concentration in humans (Isley *et al.* 1983; Clemmons *et al.* 1985). Men who adopt a vegan diet, which contains no animal protein and is therefore relatively low in essential amino acids, have been found to have a significant 9% lower IGF-I concentration compared with lacto-ovo-vegetarians and meat eaters (Allen *et al.* 2000). The lower IGF-I concentration associated with a vegan diet may be of clinical importance because differences of a similar magnitude have been found to be predictive of prostate cancer risk (Chan *et al.* 1998b). The low rates of prostate cancer found in Asian countries might therefore be partly due to dietary differences, whereby a traditional Asian diet low in animal protein may reduce IGF-I activity and hence lower prostate cancer risk.

Conclusion

Only a small proportion of prostate tumours manifest themselves clinically and most remain latent, being diagnosed incidentally during routine surgical procedures. The wide variation in prostate cancer incidence rates across the world, and the rapid increase in cancer incidence seen over recent years, can be partly explained by early detection and diagnosis of asymptomatic disease. However, the large geographical variation in mortality rates suggests that there are real differences in the incidence of clinical, aggressive disease between populations. Evidence from migrant studies suggests that both genetic and environmental factors are important in the development of clinical disease, perhaps via hormonal mechanisms.

Epidemiological evidence suggests that there may be an association between prostate cancer incidence and consumption of Western-style diets that are high in animal fat and protein and low in starchy foods, legumes and vegetables. There has been much speculation that dietary factors may affect prostate cancer development via their effects on hormone secretion and metabolism. Bioavailable androgen levels are controlled by effective homoeostasis and have not been shown to be affected by dietary factors. However, recent evidence suggests that a diet low in animal protein may reduce circulating IGF-I levels to an extent that is of biological importance in determining prostate cancer risk. More research is needed to determine the relative roles of genetic and environmental factors that determine sex hormone and IGF-I levels in men and their relation to prostate cancer risk.

Acknowledgements

We are grateful to Dr Jane Green for her useful comments in preparing the manuscript.

References

Akazaki K & Stemmerman GN (1973). Comparative study of latent carcinoma of the prostate among Japanese in Japan and Hawaii. *Journal of the National Cancer Institute* **50**, 1137–1144

Allen NE & Key TJ (2000). The effects of diet on circulating sex hormone levels in men. *Nutrition Research Reviews* **12**, 1–27

Allen NE, Appleby PN, Davey GK, Key TJ (2000). Hormones and diet: low insulin-like growth factor-I but normal bioavailable androgens in vegan men. *British Journal of Cancer* **83**, 95–97

Armstrong B & Doll R (1975). Environmental factors and cancer incidence and mortality in different countries, with special reference to dietary practices. *International Journal of Cancer* **15**, 617–631

Breslow N, Chan CW, Dhom G *et al.* (1977). Latent carcinoma of prostate of autopsy in seven areas. *International Journal of Cancer* **20**, 680–688

Brewster DH, Fraser LA, Harris V, Black RJ (2000). Rising incidence of prostate cancer in Scotland: increased risk or increased detection? *BJU International* **85**, 463–472

Carter BS, Carter HB, Isaacs JT (1990). Epidemiologic evidence regarding predisposing factors to prostate cancer. *Prostate* **16**, 187–197

Carter BS, Bova GS, Beaty TH *et al.* (1993). Hereditary prostate cancer: epidemiologic and clinical features. *Journal of Urology* **150**, 797–802

Chamberlain J, Melia J, Moss S, Brown J (1997). Report prepared for the Health Technology Assessment panel of the NHS Executive on the diagnosis, management, treatment and costs of prostate cancer in England and Wales. *British Journal of Urology* **79**, 1–32

Chan JM, Giovannucci E, Andersson SO, Yuen J, Adami HO, Wolk A (1998a). Dairy products, calcium, phosphorous, vitamin D, and risk of prostate cancer (Sweden). *Cancer Causes and Control* **9**, 559–566

Chan JM, Stampfer MJ, Giovannucci E *et al.* (1998b). Plasma insulin-like growth factor-I and prostate cancer risk: a prospective study. *Science* **279**, 563–566

Chan JM, Stampfer MJ, Ma J, Rimm EB, Willett WC, Giovannucci EL (1999). Supplemental vitamin E intake and prostate cancer risk in a large cohort of men in the United States. *Cancer Epidemiology, Biomarkers and Prevention* **8**, 893–899

Chodak GW (1994). Screening for prostate cancer: the debate continues. *Journal of the American Medical Association* **272**, 813–814

Clark LC, Combs GFJ, Turnbull BW *et al.* (1996). Effects of selenium supplementation for cancer prevention in patients with carcinoma of the skin: a randomized controlled trial. *Journal of the American Medical Association* **276**, 1957–1963

Clemmons DR, Seek MM, Underwood LE (1985). Supplemental essential amino acids augment the somatomedin-C/insulin-like growth factor-I response to re-feeding after fasting. *Metabolism Clinical and Experimental* **34**, 391–395

Connolly JM & Rose DP (1994). Regulation of DU145 human prostate cancer cell proliferation by insulin-like growth factors and its interaction with the epidermal growth factor autocrine loop. *Prostate* **24**, 167–175

Cook, PJ, Doll R, Fellingham SA (1969). A mathematical model for the age distribution of cancer in man. *International Journal of Cancer* **4**, 93–112

Crawford ED & DeAntoni EP (1993). PSA as a screening test for prostate cancer. *Urologic Clinics of North America* **20**, 637–646

Culig Z, Hobisch A, Cronauer MV *et al.* (1996). Regulation of prostatic growth and function by peptide growth factors. *Prostate* **28**, 392–405

Devgan SA, Henderson BE, Yu MC *et al.* (1997). Genetic variation of 3 beta-hydroxysteroid dehydrogenase type II in three racial/ethnic groups: implications for prostate cancer risk. *Prostate* **33**, 9–12

Eaton NE, Reeves GK, Appleby PN, Key TJ (1999). Endogenous sex hormones and prostate cancer: a quantitative review of prospective studies. *British Journal of Cancer* **80**, 930–934

Eichholzer M, Stahelin H B, Ludin E, Bernasconi F (1999). Smoking, plasma vitamins C, E, retinol, and carotene, and fatal prostate cancer: seventeen-year follow-up of the prospective basel study. *Prostate* **38**, 189–198

Etzioni R, Legler JM, Feuer EJ, Merrill RM, Cronin KA, Hankey BF (1999). Cancer surveillance series: interpreting trends in prostate cancer-part III: Quantifying the link between population prostate-specific antigen testing and recent declines in prostate cancer mortality. *Journal of the National Cancer Institute* **91**, 1033–1039

Febbo PG, Kantoff PW, Platz EA *et al.* (1999). The V89L polymorphism in the 5alpha-reductase type 2 gene and risk of prostate cancer. *Cancer Research* **59**, 5878–5881

Feuer EJ, Merrill RM, Hankey BF (1999). Cancer surveillance series: interpreting trends in prostate cancer-part II: cause of death misclassification and the recent rise and fall in prostate cancer mortality. *Journal of the National Cancer Institute* **91**, 1025–1032

Gann PH, Ma J, Giovannucci E *et al.* (1999). Lower prostate cancer risk in men with elevated plasma lycopene levels: results of a prospective analysis. *Cancer Research* **59**, 1225–1230

Giovannucci E, Ascherio A, Rimm EB, Stampfer MJ, Colditz GA, Willett WC (1995). Intake of carotenoids and retinol in relation to risk of prostate cancer. *Journal of the National Cancer Institute* **87**, 1767–1776

Giovannucci E, Stampfer MJ, Krithivas K *et al.* (1997). The CAG repeat within the androgen receptor gene and its relationship to prostate cancer. *Proceedings of the National Academy of Sciences of the USA* **94**, 3320–3323

Gohagan JK, Prorok PC, Kramer BS, Cornett JE (1994). Prostate cancer screening in the prostate, lung, colorectal and ovarian cancer screening trial of the National Cancer Institute. *Journal of Urology* **152**, 1905–1909

Grulich AE, Swerdlow AJ, dos Santos Silva I, Beral V (1995). Is the apparent rise in cancer mortality in the elderly real? Analysis of changes in certification and coding of cause of death in England and Wales, 1970-1990. *International Journal of Cancer* **63**, 164–168

Haenzel E & Hurihara M (1968). Studies of Japanese migrants I: mortality from cancer and other disease among Japanese in the U.S. *Journal of the National Cancer Institute* **40**, 43–68

Harman SM, Metter EJ, Blackman MR *et al.* (2000). Serum levels of insulin-like growth factor-I (IGF-I), IGF-II, IGF-binding protein 3 and prostate-specific antigen as predictors of clinical prostate cancer. *Journal of Clinical Endocrinology and Metabolism* **85**, 4258–4265

Heinonen OP, Albanes D, Virtamo J *et al.* (1998). Prostate cancer and supplementation with alpha-tocopherol and beta-carotene: incidence and mortality in a controlled trial. *Journal of the National Cancer Institute* **90**, 440–446

Hennekens CH, Buring JE, Manson JE *et al.* (1996). Lack of effect of long-term supplementation with beta carotene on the incidence of malignant neoplasms and cardiovascular disease. *New England Journal of Medicine* **334**, 1145–1149

IARC (1997). *Cancer Incidence in Five Continents*. Lyon, France: International Agency for Research on Cancer, World Health Organization

Ingles SA, Haile RW, Henderson BE *et al.* (1997a). Strength of linkage disequilibrium between two vitamin D receptor markers in five ethnic groups: implications for association studies. *Cancer Epidemiology Biomarkers and Prevention* **6**, 93–98

Ingles SA, Ross RK, Yu MC *et al.* (1997b). Association of prostate cancer risk with genetic polymorphisms in vitamin D receptor and androgen receptor. *Journal of the National Cancer Institute* **89**, 166–170

Isley WL, Underwood LE, Clemmons DR (1983). Dietary components that regulate serum somatomedin-C concentrations in humans. *Journal of Clinical Investigation* **71**, 175–182

Kristal AR & Cohen JH (2000). Tomatoes, lycopene, and prostate cancer. How strong is the evidence? *American Journal of Epidemiology* **151**, 124–127

Kolonel LN, Nomura AM, Cooney RV (1999). Dietary fat and prostate cancer: current status. *Journal of the National Cancer Institute* **91**, 414–428

Legler JM, Feuer EJ, Potosky AL, Merrill RM, Kramer BS (1998). The role of prostate-specific antigen (PSA). testing patterns in the recent prostate cancer incidence decline in the United States. *Cancer Causes and Control* **9**, 519–527

Lichtenstein P, Holm NV, Verkasalo PK *et al.* (2000). Environmental and heritable factors in the causation of cancer-analyses of cohorts of twins from Sweden, Denmark, and Finland. *New England Journal of Medicine* **343**, 78–85

Lunn RM, Bell DA, Mohler JL, Taylor JA (1999). Prostate cancer risk and polymorphism in 17 hydroxylase (CYP17) and steroid reductase (SRD5A2). *Carcinogenesis* **20**, 1727–1731

Makridakis NM, Ross RK, Pike MC *et al.* (1999). Association of mis-sense substitution in SRD5A2 gene with prostate cancer in African-American and Hispanic men in Los Angeles, USA. *The Lancet* **354**, 975–978

Merrill RM, Feuer EJ, Warren JL, Schussler N, Stephenson RA (1999). Role of transurethral resection of the prostate in population-based prostate cancer incidence rates. *American Journal of Epidemiology* **150**, 848–860

Messina MJ, Persky V, Setchell KD, Barnes S (1994). Soy intake and cancer risk: a review of the in vitro and in vivo data. *Nutrition and Cancer* **21**, 113–131

Mettlin C (1997). Recent developments in the epidemiology of prostate cancer. *European Journal of Cancer* **33**, 340–347

Moon TD, Brawer MK, Wilt TJ (1995). Prostate Intervention Versus Observation Trial (PIVOT): a randomized trial comparing radical prostatectomy with palliative expectant management for treatment of clinically localized prostate cancer. *Journal of the National Cancer Institute* **19**, 69–71

Moyad MA (1999). Soy, disease prevention, and prostate cancer. *Seminars in Urologic Oncology* **17**, 97–102

Noble RL (1977). The development of prostate adenocarcinoma in Nb rats following prolonged sex hormone administration. *International Review of Experimental Pathology* **23**, 113–159

Nomura AM & Kolonel LN (1991). Prostate cancer: a current perspective. *Epidemiologic Reviews* **13**, 200–227

Office for National Statistics (1984–1994). *Cancer Statistics Registrations, England and Wales,* Series MBI nos. 16–27. London: The Stationery Office

Office for National Statistics (1988–1998). *Mortality Statistics, England and Wales,* Series DH nos. 15–25. London: The Stationery Office

Office for National Statistics (2000). Registrations of cancer diagnosed in 1994–1997, England and Wales. *Health Statistics Quarterly* **7**, 71–82

Oliver SE, Gunnell D, Donovan JL (2000). Comparison of trends in prostate-cancer mortality in England and Wales and the USA. *The Lancet* **355**, 1788–1789

Omenn GS, Goodman GE, Thornquist MD *et al.* (1996). Risk factors for lung cancer and for intervention effects in CARET, the Beta-Carotene and Retinol Efficacy Trial. *Journal of the National Cancer Institute* **88**, 1550–1559

Osegbe DN (1997). Prostate cancer in Nigerians: facts and non-facts. *Journal of Urology* **157**, 1340–1343

Potosky A, Kessler L, Gridley G, Brown CC, Horm JW (1990). Rise in prostatic cancer incidence associated with increased use of transurethral resection. *Journal of the National Cancer Institute* **82**, 1624–1628

Reichardt JK, Makridakis N, Henderson BE, Yu MC, Pike MC, Ross RK (1995). Genetic variability of the human SRD5A2 gene: implications for prostate cancer risk. *Cancer Research* **55**, 3973–3975

Rittmaster RS, Zwicker H, Thompson DL, Konok G, Norman RW (1993). Androstanediol glucuronide production in human liver, prostate, and skin: evidence for the importance of the liver in 5α-reduced androgen metabolism. *Journal of Clinical Endocrinology and Metabolism* **76**, 977–982

Rohr LR (1987). Incidental adenocarcinoma in transurethral resections of the prostate: partial versus complete microscopic examination. *American Journal of Surgical Pathology* **11**, 53–58

Rose DP, Boyar AP, Wynder EL (1986). International comparisons of mortality rates for cancer of the breast, ovary, prostate, and colon, and per capita food consumption. *Cancer* **58**, 2363–2371

Schroeder FH, Damhuis RA, Kirkels WJ *et al.* (1996). European randomized study of screening for prostate cancer – the Rotterdam pilot studies. *International Journal of Cancer* **65**, 145–151

Shimizu H, Ross RK, Bernstein L (1991). Possible underestimation of the incidence rate of prostate cancer in Japan. *Japanese Journal of Cancer Research* **82**, 483–485

Stattin P, Bylund A, Rinaldi S *et al.* (2000). Plasma insulin-like growth factor-1, insulin-like growth factor-binding proteins, and prostate cancer: a prospective study. *Journal of the National Cancer Institute* **92**, 1910–1917

Thissen JP, Ketelslegers JM, Underwood LE (1994). Nutritional regulation of the insulin-like growth factors. *Endocrine Reviews* **15**, 80–101

Thomas JA (1999). Diet, micronutrients, and the prostate gland. *Nutrition Reviews* **57**, 95–103

Ward J, Young J, Sladden M (1998). Australian general practitioners' views and use of tests to detect early prostate cancer. *Australian and New Zealand Journal of Public Health* **22**, 374–380

World Health Organization (1998). *Cancer Mortality Database.* http://www.dep.iarc.fr/dataava/globocan/who.htm

World Cancer Research Fund (1997). *Nutrition and the Prevention of Cancer: A global perspective.* Washington DC: American Institute for Cancer Research

Yoshizawa K, Willett WC, Morris SJ *et al.* (1998). Study of prediagnostic selenium level in toenails and the risk of advanced prostate cancer. *Journal of the National Cancer Institute* **90**, 1219–1224

PART 2

Diagnosis

Defining the window of opportunity for curative intervention: effectiveness and efficiency in the early detection of prostate cancer and the role of case finding

Mark R Feneley and Richard Parkinson

Introduction

Curative treatment for prostate carcinoma is most reliably assured by definitive therapy of early stage disease, be it radiotherapy or surgery (D'Amico *et al.* 1998). No treatment for systemic disease achieves equivalent longterm disease-free survival. In well-selected men, radical prostatectomy offers excellent cancer control and quality of life (Walsh 2000). It is the only treatment for which outcomes can be related to pathological stage. Excellent disease-free survival is achieved in men with organ-confined disease detected by case finding, and cancer-specific outcomes correlate directly with pathological stage (Epstein *et al.* 1996). This contrasts sharply with the limited significance of similar clinical stage disease diagnosed after symptomatic presentation when prolonged survival is frequently precluded by more advanced age and unrelated co-morbidity (George 1988).

With the advent of prostate-specific antigen (PSA) testing, complementing digital rectal examination (DRE), the means of detecting prostate cancer consistently at an organ-confined stage has been established (Feneley *et al.* 2000a). This has given men the opportunity to optimise disease-specific outcome through early diagnosis and treatment. Surgical practice in centres of excellence has provided considerable further insight into the pathology of prostate cancer and the clinical behaviour of early stage disease (Walsh *et al.* 1994; Zincke *et al.* 1994; Catalona & Smith 1998).

This chapter examines how such prognostic indicators can be used to indicate potentially curable cancer and form a rational basis for patient selection.

Where may opportunities for improving prostate cancer-specific outcome be sought?

One of the fundamental difficulties in the management of early stage prostate cancer lies in the reliable identification of patients who will benefit from radical treatment (Whitmore 1973). When such therapy is being contemplated for these individuals, there are important concerns to be addressed. These include both historical enigmas that have persisted as medical doctrine and the new challenges of modern urological oncology.

Before treatment can be recommended for early stage prostate cancer, the individual patient's situation needs to be examined in relation to ideal criteria. First, the threat of the prostate cancer to the future health of the patient not only should be significant but should also be substantially reduced by the proposed treatment (Wilson & Jungner 1969). Second, the individual must be sufficiently healthy to tolerate this treatment without a medically unacceptable risk of complications, and sequelae. Finally, the patient must understand the benefits, risks and potential complications before deciding to undergo treatment. Resolving the first of these issues is likely to be the most controversial.

Clinical disease associated with prostate cancer is usually locally extensive or metastatic at symptomatic presentation. Advanced stage disease is acquired over a decade or more through progression of clinically localised tumours. In men currently diagnosed by case finding who eventually prove to have had tumours that were not cured by definitive local treatment, clinical disease may not become manifest for considerably longer (Pound *et al.* 1999). Present uncertainty focuses on two questions: for whom does radical treatment of early stage cancer prevent future clinical disease, and for whom is this worthwhile?

To address these questions, the threat of early stage prostate cancer and the benefit of treatment need to be defined. These would be determined most objectively from an outcome analysis of prospective controlled randomised trials. At the present time such trials are in place, but none has been completed (Gohagan *et al.* 1995; Schroder *et al.* 1999). Current recommendations must therefore be based on observations.

Observational data, however, may be influenced significantly by case selection. Consequently, outcomes may be biased unpredictably, particularly through effects of disease lead time and length discrepancies (Prorok *et al.* 1990). Observational comparisons nevertheless do indicate that the growth rate and capacity of early stage prostate cancer to cause clinical disease may vary considerably between different individuals with similar tumour morphology (Franks 1956). However, clinical significance is determined not only by cancer-specific factors but also by host variables, particularly survival.

It has long been recognised that disease-free survival following definitive surgical treatment is significantly disadvantaged by more advanced pathological stage, and higher tumour grade (Jewett 1980). However, because more advanced stage also confers an unfavourable lead time and length bias, it is not possible to determine the extent to which treating organ-confined cancer and achieving prolonged disease-free survival may provide a survival advantage. Although this uncertainty is of central importance in the therapeutic debate, it frequently leaves the patient seeking his advantage through cancer-free survival, believing this provides the best opportunity for cure.

The same medical controversy that questions whether or not biologically significant disease can be cured by local treatment also questions whether or not a survival advantage is gained by cure. Here, cure would be defined as disease-free survival until death. The issue underlying all these uncertainties relates to over-treatment of biologically insignificant disease. Over-treatment of early stage prostate cancer arises either from failure to recognise a cancer as biologically insignificant at diagnosis or death from causes other than prostate cancer within the natural history of the tumour. If it is conceded that cure may be worthwhile (at least in a subset of patients), it becomes essential to identify and define those aspects of the clinical disease that would indicate that cure is both achievable and necessary.

Prostate cancer accounts for over 10,000 deaths per year, and is the second most common cause of cancer death in men in the UK. These advanced and invariably metastatic tumours can be taken to have progressed over a prolonged period from biologically significant early stage disease, similar to those currently diagnosed by case finding. The benefit of treatment and subsequent disease-free survival will therefore be restricted to those individuals who had biologically significant early stage disease at diagnosis and whose life expectancy exceeds the natural history of alternatively managed clinical disease.

Definitive treatment of organ confined disease detected by case finding can achieve over 90% disease-free survival (Pound *et al.* 1997). Approximately 16% of men with non-palpable, PSA-detected cancer (stage T1c) have pathologically insignificant disease at the time of diagnosis (defined as organ-confined tumours with a Gleason Sum Score <7 and volume <0.2 ml) (Epstein *et al.* 1994). It may be reasonable therefore to anticipate that, with appropriate case selection, early treatment would benefit the majority of patients. In those for whom intervention would not be beneficial (presently, indistinguishable by pre-therapeutic criteria), the pathology would be either too advanced or would never have developed into clinical disease.

This rest of this chapter focuses on outcomes in patients treated for clinically localised prostate cancer, distinguishing those who achieve excellent disease-free survival from those who eventually develop recurrence. By identifying prognostic markers, it may be possible to develop windows of opportunity for curative treatment of prostate cancer in those situations where treatment will be most beneficial.

Predicting tumour stage and prognosis

After considering the predictable behaviour of prostate cancer, certain patients with early stage disease and a reasonable life expectancy may wish to consider undergoing radical treatment (Albertsen *et al.* 1998). For tumours diagnosed by case finding, radical prostatectomy offers an excellent probability of cure, particularly when the pathology is organ confined, and, overall, around two-thirds of patients are disease free at 10 years (Gerber *et al.* 1996; Pound *et al.* 1997). Pathological stage can be predicted by careful preoperative assessment, and clinical indices can be used to define a window of opportunity for curative intervention (Figure 3.1).

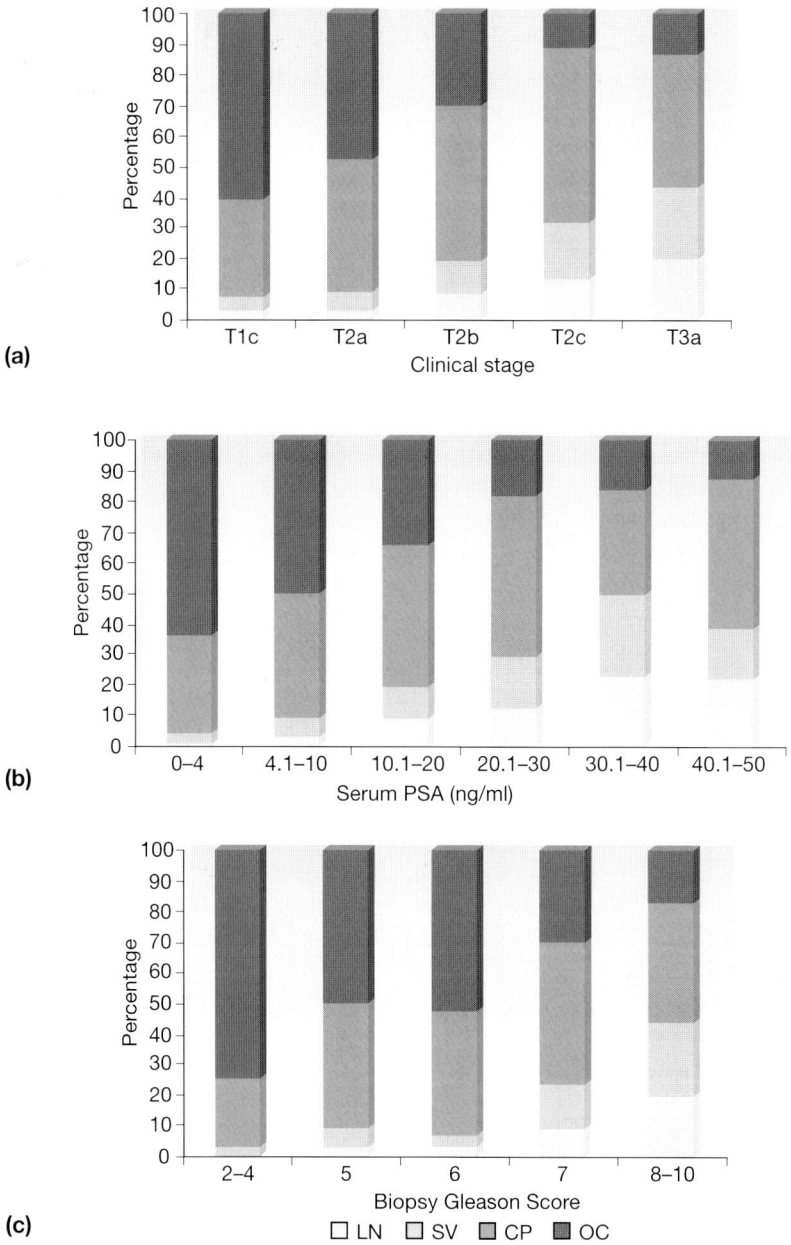

Figure 3.1 Distribution of pathological stage in men with clinically localised prostate cancer, according to (a) clinical stage (b) preoperative serum PSA level, (c) biopsy Gleason Sum Score. OC, organ confined; CP, capsular penetration; SV, seminal vesicle invasion; LN, regional lymph node metastases. Based on published data (Partin *et al.* 1997).

Clinical staging by DRE alone is notoriously unreliable, as demonstrated in patients treated by radical prostatectomy. Although DRE is a significant independent predictor of eventual pathological stage (Partin *et al.* 1997), palpable tumours that are clinically organ confined are more likely to be extracapsular on pathological staging than tumours detected by PSA alone (Ramos *et al.* 1999). DRE therefore has a poor negative predictive value for extraprostatic disease, which is recognised to be associated with a significantly greater risk of disease recurrence after definitive therapy (Chodak *et al.* 1989; O'Dowd *et al.* 1997).

Although serum PSA elevation is not specific for the presence of prostate cancer, levels broadly correlate with the likelihood of malignancy (Stamey *et al.* 1987; Oesterling 1991). It is well established that most non-palpable tumours detected by PSA meet volume and grade criteria to be classified as pathologically significant (Stamey *et al.* 1989; Epstein *et al.* 1994). Attempts to improve the clinical effectiveness of PSA include correction for gland volume (PSA density) (Benson *et al.* 1992; Catalona *et al.* 1994b), age-specific reference ranges (Dalkin *et al.* 1995; Oesterling *et al.* 1993), determination of PSA velocity (Keetch *et al.* 1996; Carter *et al.* 1997a), and comparison of different molecular forms of PSA (Catalona *et al.* 1995; Epstein *et al.* 1998). Although these modifications may improve specificity, this is frequently at the expense of sensitivity, raising concerns that failure to biopsy may compromise the chance of successful curative treatment for individuals with cancer. These parameters may also indicate the likelihood of cancer missed on initial biopsy, and the need for more frequent biopsy on follow-up of abnormal test results (Feneley *et al.* 1995a; Ukimura *et al.* 1997).

In men already diagnosed with prostate cancer, PSA levels correlate directly with pathological stage (Catalona *et al.* 1993; Partin *et al.* 1997) and recurrence rates ensuing after treatment (Stamey *et al.* 1989). Thus, PSA values significantly greater than 10.0 ng/ml are more frequently associated with extracapsular extension (Partin *et al.* 1997). Of men with PSA-detected cancers (stage T1c), around one-third having radical prostatectomy prove to have extracapsular tumour at pathological examination (Epstein *et al.* 1994). PSA cut-offs alone, however, do not distinguish tumours that are pathologically organ confined sufficiently reliably in the individual patient (Stamey *et al.* 1989; Partin *et al.* 1990, 1997).

Surgical series have demonstrated the importance of tumour grade in relation to therapeutic outcome. Historical observations in untreated men demonstrate that very well-differentiated malignancy is rarely life-threatening with short- to medium-term follow-up (Johansson *et al.* 1992; Chodak *et al.* 1994). Gleason Sum Score 2–4 invariably indicates low malignant potential (Albertsen *et al.* 1998) and these tumours are uncommonly diagnosed on needle biopsy, because they occur predominantly in the transition zone (Greene *et al.* 1991). Significant tumours seem to be reliably detected by systematic needle biopsy, provided the far lateral peripheral zone is adequately sampled (Chang *et al.* 1998a; Eskew *et al.* 1998). Transition zone biopsies have been shown to be most worthwhile in men with peripheral zone biopsies negative for tumour (Fleshner & Fair 1997) and in men with larger prostates (>50 ml) (Chang *et al.* 1998b). The multifocality of tumours detected by needle biopsy may only be appreciated fully in men having radical prostatectomy (Byar & Mostofi 1972; Epstein & Steinberg 1990).

Gleason sum score of preoperative biopsies is predictive of pathological stage (Partin *et al.* 1997) and tumour recurrence (Pound *et al.* 1997). Sum Scores of 8–10 have been associated with a probability of non-organ-confined disease and recurrence at 10 years of over 80% (Pound *et al.* 1997). However, in men whose biopsies show less poorly differentiated cancer, sampling error associated with under-grading may occur in as many as 30% (Epstein & Steinberg 1990). Increasing the number of biopsy cores and repeat biopsy may be necessary to improve diagnostic accuracy. The majority of men undergoing radical prostatectomy have moderately differentiated tumours and, in these individuals, grade alone contributes to prediction of pathological stage in fewer than 15% after taking DRE and PSA findings into consideration (Partin *et al.* 1993).

The combined use of DRE, PSA and Gleason Score is much more powerful in the preoperative staging of prostate cancer than any one of these indices alone. Nomograms that relate clinical stage, Gleason Score and PSA to pathological stage have been published (Partin *et al.* 1993) and their use validated in a multi-institutional study (Figure 3.2) (Partin *et al.* 1997). These can be used to predict pathological stage from preoperative variables, and their use in clinical decision-

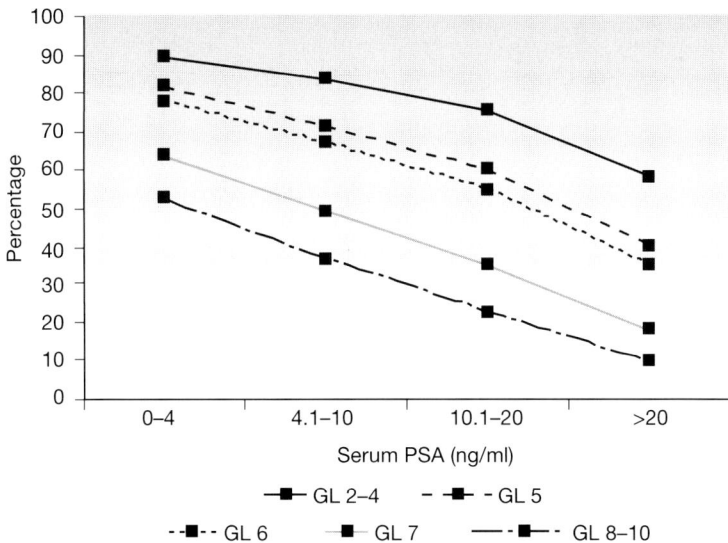

Figure 3.2 Probability of pathologically organ-confined cancer according to serum PSA and biopsy Gleason Sum Score in men with PSA-detected cancer (stage T1c) Based on published data (Partin *et al.* 1997).

making has been corroborated in a pre-radiation setting as well (Roach *et al.* 1994). Further use of nomograms predicting disease recurrence after radical prostatectomy has been proposed. Some incorporate pathological stage, restricting their use to men treated surgically (Kattan *et al.* 1999) and others are based entirely on preoperative indices, extending their potential clinical application (Kattan *et al.* 1998).

In men with non-palpable prostate cancer (stage T1c), those individuals most likely to develop disease recurrence after treatment may be identified quite simply by a combination of preoperative PSA and biopsy Gleason Sum Score (Feneley & Partin 2001). Cut-offs can be established by the receiver operating characteristics of the two variables. In a retrospective analysis, PSA <12 ng/ml combined with Gleason Sum Score <7 was associated with an extremely high probability of long-term PSA-free survival after local radical surgery. Biochemical recurrence was significantly greater in men with PSA levels over 12 ng/ml or Gleason Sum Score ≥7. Since this may represent an important means of subdividing stage T1c into stages $T1c_I$ and $T1c_{II}$ for prognostic discrimination, prospective validation is essential (Figure 3.3).

Biopsy provides valuable information other than grade which may be independently valuable for predicting pathological stage and prognosis. A relationship between perineural invasion in biopsy specimens and pathological stage has been suggested (de la Taille *et al.* 1999), but is not universally accepted (Egan & Bostwick 1997; Holmes *et al.* 1999). Prognostic information appears to be gained from the percentage of cores involved (Ravery *et al.* 1994; Presti *et al.* 1998), microvessel density (Bostwick *et al.* 1996; Silberman *et al.* 1997), DNA ploidy (Badalament *et al.* 1996;

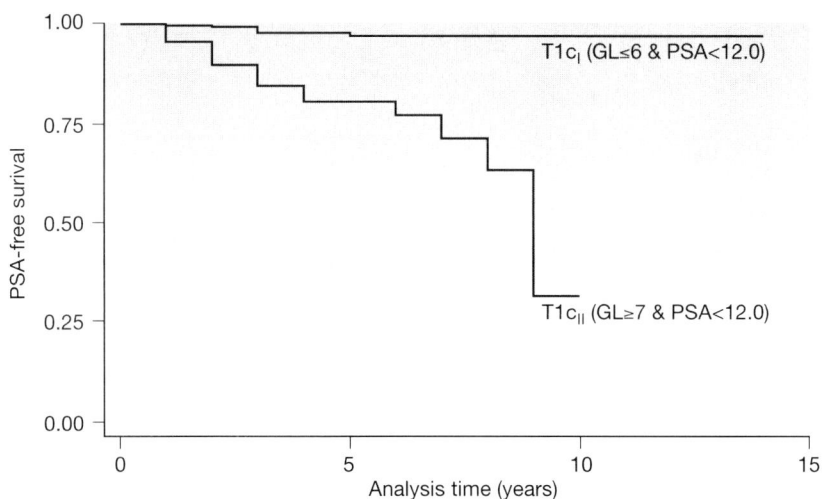

Figure 3.3 Kaplan–Meier actuarial survival estimates for patients with stage T1c prostate cancer according to proposed substaging by biopsy Gleason Score (GL) and preoperative PSA. Based on data (M Feneley, unpublished data).

Veltri *et al.* 1998) and various biomarkers (Scherr *et al.* 1999). Biomarkers of particular interest include p53 mutations, increased expression of *bcl*-2, and decreased expression of E-cadherin and *KAI*-1. Their place in routine clinical practice is yet to be established.

Defining the window for cure?

The word 'cure' can be variously defined as 'to get rid of an ailment' or 'to restore to health'. We will consider a curative treatment to be one that results in the patient being permanently free of cancer. At present, the lack of effective systemic treatments for metastatic or locally advanced cancers means that curative treatment for prostate carcinoma is most reliably assured for patients with pathologically organ-confined disease.

Radical prostatectomy represents the most definitive treatment for organ-confined prostate cancer. Historically, its popularity has been limited by complications, including bleeding, impotence, urinary incontinence and anastomotic strictures. Following description of the anatomical basis of the surgical approach to prostatectomy by Walsh, low operative morbidity can be achieved without compromising cancer cure (Walsh 1998).

Before the advent of PSA testing, reliance on DRE in the preoperative assessment of prostate cancers was associated with a high rate of understaging. Around half of palpable but clinically organ-confined tumours proved to be more advanced at prostatectomy (Chodak *et al.* 1989). PSA is arguably the best of all serum tumour markers and provides the means by which prostate cancer can be diagnosed at an early and curable stage (Catalona *et al.* 1993), with an estimated lead time of approximately 5 years (Gann *et al.* 1995). In countries where men have been exposed to testing, there has been a significant stage shift towards lower stage disease at diagnosis, and there have been encouraging observations consistent with improved cancer-specific outcome (Gilliland *et al.* 1994; Farkas *et al.* 1998).

Population screening with DRE and PSA has been shown to be feasible, both in the USA and in the UK. Cancer detection rates of between 1.5% and 6% are most commonly observed (Chodak *et al.* 1989; Brewster *et al.* 1994; Catalona *et al.* 1994a; Feneley *et al.* 1995a). However, in both countries, substantially higher detection rates (15–29%) have been observed when case finding is undertaken in an outpatient urological practice (Cooner *et al.* 1990; Feneley 1999). Differences in age, the presence of symptoms and abnormal test results in patients referred for urological evaluation may be expected to contribute to a higher prevalence of cancer than would be observed in an asymptomatic screened population. Indeed, as a result of case finding, the prevalence of symptoms in men undergoing radical prostatectomy in the USA is substantially lower now than it was in the pre-PSA era (Gilliland *et al.* 1994).

In the setting of case finding, detection rates for prostate cancer and stage distribution will be influenced significantly by demographic characteristics of the tested population, as well as prior exposure to testing, distribution of abnormal tests and criteria used for biopsy. The accuracy of the tests themselves can be determined only when the true prevalence of cancer in the study population is known. This includes not only cancers detected by abnormal test results, but also those that were missed – either because of a false-negative biopsy or because of false-negative test results.

A study, performed at St Bartholomew's Hospital, London, examined the performance of PSA and DRE for predicting cancer on needle biopsy (Feneley 1999). Referred patients without suspicion of extraprostatic invasion by malignant disease had sextant prostate biopsies irrespective of PSA and DRE test results. The findings confirmed the value of combining both DRE and PSA in a cancer detection program. In 105 patients, (age range 50–76, median 67 years), 26 (25%) had abnormal DRE, 54 (51%) had PSA greater than 4.0 ng/ml and 30 (29%) had cancer. The accuracy of DRE and PSA for predicting cancer is described in Table 3.1. For therapeutic purposes, however, it is necessary to distinguish those cancers that are *both* curable by radical treatment *and* not insignificant by pathological criteria at the time of diagnosis.

Table 3.1 Performance of screening tests (DRE and PSA) for predicting cancer on systematic prostatic biopsy in a population of 105 men referred with no evidence of extraprostatic malignancy. All men had prostate biopsy irrespective of prior screening test results. Based on published data (Feneley 1999)

	Digital rectal examination (%)	Serum PSA (cut-off >4.0 ng/ml) (%)
Positive predictive value	54	41
Negative predictive value	80	84
Sensitivity	47	73
Specificity	84	57

Both the likelihood of non-curable cancer and that of insignificant cancer can be predicted from indices provided by careful clinical evaluation. The Partin tables, discussed previously, provide important criteria-based prediction of pathological stage, including reliability of the prediction with confidence intervals, based on multi-institutional data (Partin *et al.* 1997).

The presence of pathologically insignificant cancer at diagnosis can also be inferred from clinical indices. In a single centre observational setting, the combination of PSA density <0.15 ng/ml per g, biopsy Gleason pattern <3, fewer than three cores involved with cancer, and less than 50% involvement of any core have been shown to be strongly predictive of insignificant cancer (defined as smaller than 0.2 ml, Gleason Sum Score <7 and organ confined) (Epstein *et al.* 1994). In prospective evaluation of 240 men with stage T1c tumours treated by radical prostatectomy, 75% of those fulfilling these preoperative criteria had either insignificant or minimal disease, compared to 16% of those who did not fulfil these criteria (Carter *et al.* 1997b). In a subsequent analysis of 144 men who met the same criteria for insignificant disease and were managed expectantly for 0–6 years, unfavourable histology (i.e. no longer meeting the above criteria) was eventually demonstrated at annual biopsy in 25%, and considered to represent progression (Carter *et al.* 2000). Of those who then elected for radical prostatectomy, two-thirds were considered to have curable tumours. In the one-third who had more advanced tumour, the important issue relates to the possibility of under-sampling at the time of initial biopsy. However, conservative management was feasible for most men who had favourable biopsy findings at initial biopsy. In the majority of those with subsequently unfavourable biopsy findings, cure did not seem to have been compromised by delayed treatment.

Some authors have suggested that use of PSA cut-offs below 4.0 ng/ml should be recommended on the basis of superior sensitivity, either based on age-stratified reference ranges or irrespective of age (Catalona *et al.* 1999). The prevalence of pathologically insignificant disease does not seem to be increased significantly by adopting this policy. This policy does, however, substantially increase the total number of biopsies per cancer detected, as well as anxiety and invasive testing for individuals without cancer. The number of non-palpable tumours that will no longer be organ confined when the PSA reaches 4.0 ng/ml may not justify exposing an additional very large number of men to biopsies (Carter *et al.* 1997). The underlying issue relates to the proportion of non-palpable tumours associated with PSA < 4.0 ng/ml that represent a risk to life expectancy and would no longer be curable if treatment were delayed until the PSA reached 4.0 ng/ml. This merits further consideration.

Recent evidence suggests that the PSA level may select men for biopsy according to prostate size. Review of prostate volume in men treated for organ-confined cancer by radical prostatectomy at the Johns Hopkins Hospital indicates that gland volume has increased significantly since the introduction of PSA testing (Feneley *et al.* 2000b). This is substantial in men with PSA-detected (stage T1c) disease and minimal in men with palpable (stage T2) disease (Figure 3.4). Furthermore, there was no significant difference in prostate volume in men treated before PSA testing and men without cancer. This suggests that the detection of cancer by PSA may be serendipitous in men with larger prostates, perhaps due to PSA elevation associated with benign prostatic hyperplasia (BPH).

If PSA elevation preferentially detects cancer in men with larger prostates, as this last study suggests, higher PSA cut-offs would be expected to exaggerate the bias. Lower PSA cut-offs, on the other hand, may detect cancer earlier by permitting biopsies in smaller prostates rather than by reducing the threshold for tumour-specific PSA elevation. A further analysis of the data provided by the biopsy study performed at St Bartholomew's hospital (referred to above) was therefore conducted.

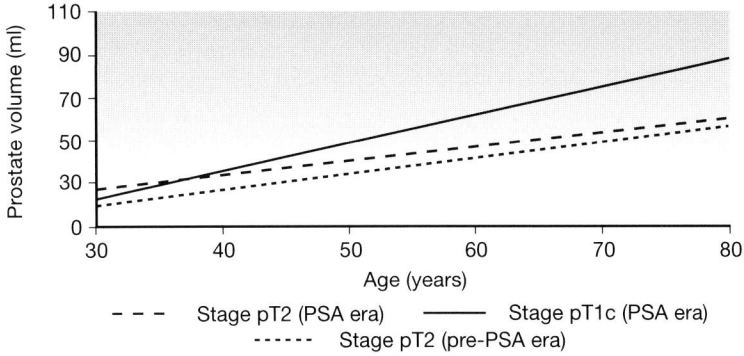

Figure 3.4 Prostate volumes in relationship to age in men undergoing radical prostatectomy for organ-confined prostate cancer in the pre-PSA era and PSA era. Tumours treated in the PSA era are subdivided into stages T1c (PSA-detected) and T2b (palpable). Based on published data (Feneley *et al.* 2000b).

This showed that in men with cancer and normal volume-adjusted PSA level, uncorrected serum PSA correlated with gland volume (Figure 3.5) (Feneley *et al.* 2000a).

Men younger than 50 years of age more frequently have curable disease than older men (Carter *et al.* 1999). Earlier age of onset of screening may therefore be a more logical approach to the detection of curable and significant tumours than lower PSA cut-offs. Although the optimal age to commence screening and subsequent

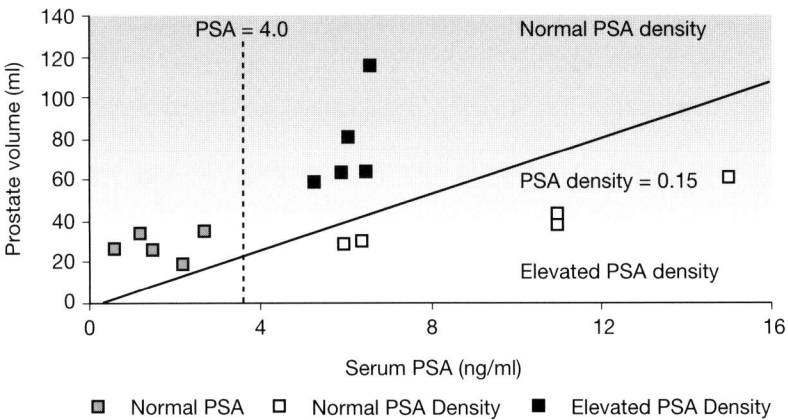

Figure 3.5 Prostate volumes and serum PSA in a men with biopsy-proven, non-palpable cancer (stage T1c) in a population undergoing systematic prostate biopsy irrespective of PSA level and DRE findings. Among those with normal volume corrected PSA (PSA density), serum PSA levels are correlated with prostate volume.

screening interval for detecting curable, significant tumours remains unproven, further research may allow recommendations based on risk. A recent observation suggests that annual follow-up may be unnecessary in men with normal DRE and PSA levels less than 2.0 ng/ml because these individuals are at very low risk of developing a significant cancer within 2 years (Carter *et al.* 1997). Furthermore, PSA levels between 2.0 ng/ml and 4.0 ng/ml may identify men most at risk of having significant (curable) stage T1c tumours if the PSA reaches 4.0 ng/ml. More frequent monitoring may also be indicated by indices other than total PSA, such as density, slope and free/total ratio, as it is in men who have already had negative biopsies (Borboroglu *et al.* 2000).

Markov modelling has been used to compare alternative prostate cancer screening strategies according to the predicted number of prostate cancer deaths prevented (Ross *et al.* 2000). This approach offers a theoretical basis for evaluating age of onset of screening, PSA threshold and screening interval in relation to outcome, which would probably not be feasible in a clinical trial setting. It uses validated estimates of age-related tumour progression rates determined from postmortem studies and tumour-related outcomes after radical prostatectomy. The analysis shows that adopting PSA levels lower than 4.0 ng/ml does not substantially improve outcome, compared with the current recommendations for screening annually from the age of 50 years. The model also demonstrates that, by commencing screening at 40 years of age, re-screening at 45 years of age and every 2 years from the age of 50, a substantially smaller number of screening tests would be required to save the same number of lives. This approach may be particularly useful where the benefit of screening is accepted.

Currently, the lack of data from well-organised randomised controlled trials of screening with PSA has confounded attempts to make evidence-based policy. Trials of screening and early treatment are in place, although, while their outcomes are awaited with interest, significant advances in diagnosis and prognostication may be achieved. By the nature of localised prostate cancer, randomised trials require a long period of follow-up (at least 10 years) before any benefit becomes manifest. Their usefulness may become limited by difficulty in defining a population not exposed to screening tests outside the influence of the study protocol (negative control), e.g. by presenting with lower urinary tract symptoms, or anxiety about the possibility of undiagnosed cancer. 'Back-door' screening such as this may become a significant source bias in the results of these trials.

The American Cancer Society and the American Urological Association recommend an annual DRE and PSA for men over 50 years of age with a life expectancy of at least 10 years, and for men over 40 with a strong family history of prostate cancer. PSA testing provides an opportunity to establish the diagnosis of prostate cancer before the onset of symptoms, and at a stage when the majority of clinically organ-confined cancers can be cured. It will result in both a stage shift and an age shift in the presentation of disease. A screened population is therefore more likely to be suitable for radical prostatectomy and have sufficient life expectancy to reap the benefit of curative treatment.

Complications of treatment: acceptability of risk and outcome

Treatment of early stage prostate cancer by surgery or radiation is likely to be associated with some degree of therapeutic morbidity. Many studies have shown that this is substantially lower in referral centres that have acquired large experience and expertise. Although cancer-specific benefit may not be gained for several years, morbidity and complications of treatment may impact on the patient more immediately and before that of untreated disease.

The alternative therapeutic options for early stage prostate cancer differ substantially in their mechanism of tumour control. The pattern of complications, their timing and eventual outcome also differ significantly. It is important that both disease and therapeutic sequelae are considered by the patient, because their acceptability is likely to influence significantly the eventual choice of therapy. Outcomes following treatment are discussed in detail elsewhere in this volume.

Conclusion

Our understanding of early stage prostate cancer has grown considerably within the last decade. In communities not exposed to screening, symptomatic presentation of prostate cancer is usually associated with advanced or metastatic (incurable) disease. Most of these patients die from their disease, accounting for the second most common cause of cancer death in men. The remainder, diagnosed with clinically localised cancer, predominantly represents elderly men who are unlikely to die from their disease.

Case-finding strategies identify men with early stage prostate cancer for whom treatment offers an excellent probability of long-term disease-free survival. Without treatment, these individuals would be at medium- or long-term risk of pathological disease progression to symptomatic, incurable disease. The eventual impact of any policy for management of early prostate cancer on population mortality is not likely to be appreciated within the natural history of these tumours (perhaps as long as 20 years). Furthermore, trends would not stabilise while a pool of incurable disease exists within the community and diagnostic techniques continue to evolve. Case finding is likely to be most effective when undertaken regularly and begun sufficiently early in a population setting.

For the individual, prostate cancer is most likely to be curable when organ- confined (pT1 and pT2). Patient selection using preoperative indices, including clinical stage, serum PSA, and Gleason grade of biopsies, identifies individuals most likely to have organ-confined disease and low risk of recurrence. It may also become possible to predict more reliably the pathological insignificance of diagnosed tumours. Patient age and co-morbidity distinguishes those for whom radical therapy may not be beneficial, but for those having early treatment, the survival benefit is as yet unproven. When considering alternative management options, the patient should understand the risks and complications of both disease and its treatment.

It is essential for future health policy to identify those positions that will provide the best opportunities for future progress. Patients may require guidelines to aid informed decisions particularly when a need for treatment is recognised and evidence of survival benefit is lacking. Evolving policies must recognise the need to ensure that individuals, wishing to present themselves for case finding, do so within evidence-based windows of opportunity shown to achieve the best outcomes from currently available therapy. The choice may be life saving.

References

Albertsen PC, Hanley JA, Gleason DF, Barry MJ (1998). Competing risk analysis of men aged 55 to 74 years at diagnosis managed conservatively for clinically localized prostate cancer. *Journal of the American Medical Association* **280**, 975–980

Badalament RA, Miller MC, Peller PA *et al.* (1996). An algorithm for predicting nonorgan confined prostate cancer using the results obtained from sextant core biopsies with prostate specific antigen level. *Journal of Urology* **156**, 1375–1380

Benson MC, Whang IS, Pantuck A *et al.* (1992). Prostate specific antigen density: a means of distinguishing benign prostatic hypertrophy and prostate cancer. *Journal of Urology* **147**, 815–816

Borboroglu PG, Comer SW, Riffenburgh RH, Amling CL (2000). Extensive repeat transrectal ultrasound guided prostate biopsy in patients with previous benign sextant biopsies. *Journal of Urology* **163**, 158–162

Bostwick DG, Wheeler TM, Blute M *et al.* (1996). Optimized microvessel density analysis improves prediction of cancer stage from prostate needle biopsies. *Urology* **48**, 47–57

Brewster SF, Kemple T, MacIver AG, Astley JP, Gingell JC (1994). The Bristol prostate cancer pilot screening study – a 3-year follow-up. *British Journal of Urology* **74**, 556–558

Byar DP & Mostofi FK (1972). Carcinoma of the prostate: prognostic evaluation of certain pathologic features in 208 radical prostatectomies. Examined by the step-section technique. *Cancer* **30**, 5–13

Carter HB & Pearson JD (1997). Prostate-specific antigen velocity and repeated measures of prostate-specific antigen. *Urologic Clinics of North America* **24**, 333–338

Carter HB, Epstein JI, Chan DW, Fozard JL, Pearson JD (1997a). Recommended prostate-specific antigen testing intervals for the detection of curable prostate cancer. *Journal of the American Medical Association* **277**, 1456–1460

Carter HB, Sauvageot J, Walsh PC, Epstein JI (1997b). Prospective evaluation of men with stage T1C adenocarcinoma of the prostate. *Journal of Urology* **157**, 2206–2209

Carter, HB, Epstein, JI, Partin, AW (1999). Influence of age and prostate-specific antigen on the chance of curable prostate cancer among men with nonpalpable disease. *Urology* **53**, 126–130

Carter HB, Landis PK, Epstein JI, Walsh PC (2000). Expectant management of prostate cancer with curative intent. *Journal of Urology* **163**, 335

Catalona WJ & Smith DS (1998). Cancer recurrence and survival rates after anatomic radical retropubic prostatectomy for prostate cancer: intermediate-term results. *Journal of Urology* **160**, 2428–2434

Catalona WJ, Smith DS, Ratliff TL, Basler JW (1993). Detection of organ-confined prostate cancer is increased through prostate-specific antigen-based screening. *Journal of the American Medical Association* **270**, 948–954

Catalona WJ, Richie JP, Ahmann FR *et al.* (1994a). Comparison of digital rectal examination and serum prostate specific antigen in the early detection of prostate cancer: results of a multicenter clinical trial of 6,630 men. *Journal of Urology* **151**, 1283–1290

Catalona WJ, Richie JP, DeKernion JB *et al.* (1994b). Comparison of prostate specific antigen concentration versus prostate specific antigen density in the early detection of prostate cancer: receiver operating characteristic curves. *Journal of Urology* **152**, 2031–2036

Catalona WJ, Smith DS, Wolfert RL *et al.* (1995). Evaluation of percentage of free serum prostate-specific antigen to improve specificity of prostate cancer screening. *Journal of the American Medical Association* **274**, 1214–1220

Catalona WJ, Partin AW, Finlay JA *et al.* (1999). Use of percentage of free prostate-specific antigen to identify men at high risk of prostate cancer when PSA levels are 2.51 to 4 ng/mL and digital rectal examination is not suspicious for prostate cancer: an alternative model. *Urology* **54**, 220–224

Chang JJ, Shinohara K, Bhargava V, Presti JCJ (1998a). Prospective evaluation of lateral biopsies of the peripheral zone for prostate cancer detection. *Journal of Urology* **160**, 2111–2114

Chang JJ, Shinohara K, Hovey RM, Montgomery C, Presti JCJ (1998b). Prospective evaluation of systematic sextant transition zone biopsies in large prostates for cancer detection. *Urology* **52**, 89–93

Chodak GW, Keller P, Schoenberg HW (1989). Assessment of screening for prostate cancer using the digital rectal examination. *Journal of Urology* **141**, 1136–1138

Chodak GW, Thisted RA, Gerber GS *et al.* (1994). Results of conservative management of clinically localized prostate cancer. *New England Journal of Medicine* **330**, 242–248

Cooner WH, Mosley BR, Rutherford CL Jr *et al.* (1990). Prostate cancer detection in a clinical urological practice by ultrasonography, digital rectal examination and prostate specific antigen. *Journal of Urology* **143**, 1146–1152

D'Amico AV, Whittington R, Malkowicz SB *et al.* (1998). Biochemical outcome after radical prostatectomy, external beam radiation therapy, or interstitial radiation therapy for clinically localized prostate cancer [see comments]. *Journal of the American Medical Association* **280**, 969–974

Dalkin BL, Ahmann FR, Kopp JB *et al.* (1995). Derivation and application of upper limits for prostate specific antigen in men aged 50–74 years with no clinical evidence of prostatic carcinoma. *British Journal of Urology* **76**, 346–350

de la Taille A, Katz A, Bagiella E, Olsson CA, O'Toole KM, Rubin MA (1999). Perineural invasion on prostate needle biopsy: an independent predictor of final pathologic stage. *Urology* **54**, 1039–1043

Egan AJ & Bostwick DG (1997). Prediction of extraprostatic extension of prostate cancer based on needle biopsy findings: perineural invasion lacks significance on multivariate analysis. *American Journal of Surgical Pathology* **21**, 1496–1500

Epstein JI & Steinberg GD (1990). The significance of low-grade prostate cancer on needle biopsy. A radical prostatectomy study of tumor grade, volume, and stage of the biopsied and multifocal tumor. *Cancer* **66**, 1927–1932

Epstein JI, Walsh PC, Carmichael M, Brendler CB (1994). Pathologic and clinical findings to predict tumor extent of nonpalpable (stage T1c) prostate cancer. *Journal of the American Medical Association* **271**, 368–374

Epstein JI, Partin AW, Sauvageot J, Walsh PC (1996). Prediction of progression following radical prostatectomy. A multivariate analysis of 721 men with long-term follow-up. *American Journal of Surgical Pathology* **20**, 286–292

Epstein JI, Chan DW, Sokoll LJ *et al.* (1998). Nonpalpable stage T1c prostate cancer: prediction of insignificant disease using free/total prostate specific antigen levels and needle biopsy findings. *Journal of Urology* **160**, 2407–2411

Eskew LA, Woodruff RD, Bare RL, McCullough DL (1998). Prostate cancer diagnosed by the 5 region biopsy method is significant disease. *Journal of Urology* **160**, 794–796

Farkas A, Schneider D, Perrotti M, Cummings KB, Ward WS (1998). National trends in the epidemiology of prostate cancer, 1973 to 1994: evidence for the effectiveness of prostate-specific antigen screening. *Urology* **52**, 444–448

Feneley MR (1999). Does screening for prostate cancer identify clinically important disease? *Annals of the Royal College of Surgeons of England* **81**, 207–214

Feneley MR & Partin AW (2000). Diagnosis of localized prostate cancer: 10 years of progress. *Current Opinion in Urology* **10**, 319–327

Feneley MR & Partin AW (2001). PSA and radical prostatectomy. In: Brawer MK (ed.) *Prostate Specific Antigen.* New York: Marcel Dekker Inc.

Feneley MR, Kirby MG, McNicholas T, McLean A, Webb JAW, Kirby RS (1995a). Screening for carcinoma of the prostate in general practice. *Cancer Surveys* **23**, 115–125

Feneley MR, Webb JA, McLean A, Kirby RS (1995b). Post-operative serial prostate-specific antigen and transrectal ultrasound for staging incidental carcinoma of the prostate. *British Journal of Urology* **75**, 14–20

Feneley MR, Holmes K, Corrie D, Kirby RS (2000a). PSA screening for impalpable prostate cancer: are biopsies driven by cancer or BPH? *BJU International* **85**, P6

Feneley MR, Landis P, Simon I *et al.* (2000b). Today men with prostate cancer have larger prostates. *Urology* **56**, 839–842

Fleshner NE & Fair WR (1997). Indications for transition zone biopsy in the detection of prostatic carcinoma. *Journal of Urology* **157**, 556–558

Franks LM (1956). The natural history of prostatic cancer. *The Lancet* **ii**, 1037–1039

Gann PH, Hennekens CH, Stampfer MJ (1995). A prospective evaluation of plasma prostate-specific antigen for detection of prostatic cancer. *Journal of the American Medical Association* **273**, 289–294

George NJR (1988). Natural history of localised prostate cancer managed by conservative therapy alone. *The Lancet* **i**, 494–497

Gerber GS, Thisted RA, Scardino PT *et al.* (1996). Results of radical prostatectomy in men with clinically localized prostate cancer. *Journal of the American Medical Association* **276**, 615–619

Gilliland F, Becker TM, Smith A, Key CR, Samet JM (1994). Trends in prostate cancer incidence and mortality in New Mexico are consistent with an increase in effective screening. *Cancer Epidemiology, Biomarkers and Prevention* **3**, 105–111

Gohagan JK, Prorok PC, Kramer BS, Hayes RB, Cornett, JE (1995). The Prostate, Lung, Colorectal, and Ovarian Cancer Screening Trial of the National Cancer Institute. *Cancer* **75**, 1869–1873

Greene DR, Wheeler TM, Egawa S, Dunn JK, Scardino PT (1991). A comparison of the morphological features of cancer arising in the transition zone and in the peripheral zone of the prostate. *Journal of Urology* **146**, 1069–1076

Holmes GF, Walsh PC, Pound CR, Epstein JI (1999). Excision of the neurovascular bundle at radical prostatectomy in cases with perineural invasion on needle biopsy. *Urology* **53**, 752–756

Jewett HJ (1980). Radical perineal prostatectomy for palpable, clinically localized, non- obstructive cancer: experience at the Johns Hopkins Hospital 1909–1963. *Journal of Urology* **124**, 492–494

Johansson JE, Adami HO, Andersson SO, Bergstrom R, Holmberg L, Krusemo UB (1992). High 10-year survival rate in patients with early, untreated prostatic cancer. *Journal of the American Medical Association* **267**, 2191–2196

Kattan MW, Eastham JA, Stapleton AM, Wheeler TM, Scardino PT (1998). A preoperative nomogram for disease recurrence following radical prostatectomy for prostate cancer. *Journal of the National Cancer Institute* **90**, 766–771

Kattan MW, Wheeler TM, Scardino PT (1999). Postoperative nomogram for disease recurrence after radical prostatectomy for prostate cancer. *Journal of Clinical Oncology* **17**, 1499–1507

Keetch DW, McMurtry JM, Smith DS, Andriole GL, Catalona WJ (1996). Prostate specific antigen density versus prostate specific antigen slope as predictors of prostate cancer in men with initially negative prostatic biopsies. *Journal of Urology* **156**, 428–431

O'Dowd GJ, Veltri RW, Orozco R, Miller MC, Oesterling JE (1997). Update on the appropriate staging evaluation for newly diagnosed prostate cancer. *Journal of Urology* **158**, 687–698

Oesterling JE (1991). Prostate specific antigen: a critical assessment of the most useful tumor marker for adenocarcinoma of the prostate. *Journal of Urology* **145**, 907–923

Oesterling JE, Jacobsen SJ, Chute CG *et al.* (1993). Serum prostate-specific antigen in a community-based population of healthy men. Establishment of age-specific reference ranges. *Journal of the American Medical Association* **270**, 860–864

Partin AW, Carter HB, Chan DW *et al.* (1990). Prostate specific antigen in the staging of localized prostate cancer: influence of tumor differentiation, tumor volume and benign hyperplasia. *Journal of Urology* **143**, 747–752

Partin AW, Yoo J, Carter HB *et al.* (1993). The use of prostate specific antigen, clinical stage and Gleason score to predict pathological stage in men with localized prostate cancer. *Journal of Urology* **150**, 110–114

Partin AW, Kattan MW, Subong EN *et al.* (1997). Combination of prostate-specific antigen, clinical stage, and Gleason score to predict pathological stage of localized prostate cancer. A multi-institutional update. *Journal of the American Medical Association* **277**, 1445–1451

Pound CR, Partin AW, Epstein JI, Walsh PC (1997). Prostate-specific antigen after anatomic radical retropubic prostatectomy. Patterns of recurrence and cancer control. *Urologic Clinics of North America* **24**, 395–406

Pound CR, Partin AW, Eisenberger MA, Chan DW, Pearson JD, Walsh PC (1999). Natural history of progression after PSA elevation following radical prostatectomy. *Journal of the American Medical Association* **281**, 1591–1597

Presti JCJ, Shinohara K, Bacchetti P, Tigrani V, Bhargava V (1998). Positive fraction of systematic biopsies predicts risk of relapse after radical prostatectomy. *Urology* **52**, 1079–1084

Prorok PC, Connor RJ, Baker SG (1990). Statistical considerations in cancer screening programs. *Urologic Clinics of North America* **17**, 699–708

Ramos CG, Carvalhal GF, Smith DS, Mager DE, Catalona WJ (1999). Clinical and pathological characteristics, and recurrence rates of stage T1c versus T2a or T2b prostate cancer. *Journal of Urology* **161**, 1525–1529

Ravery V, Boccon-Gibod LA, Dauge-Geffroy MC *et al.* (1994). Systematic biopsies accurately predict extracapsular extension of prostate cancer and persistent/recurrent detectable PSA after radical prostatectomy. *Urology* **44**, 371–376

Roach M, Marquez C, Yuo HS *et al.* (1994). Predicting the risk of lymph node involvement using the pre-treatment prostate specific antigen and Gleason score in men with clinically localized prostate cancer. *International Journal of Radiation Oncology, Biology, Physics* **28**, 33–37

Ross KS, Carter HB, Pearson JD, Guess HA (2000). Comparative efficiency of prostate-specific antigen screening strategies for prostate cancer detection. *Journal of the American Medical Association* **284**, 1399–1405

Scherr DS, Vaughan EDJ, Wei J *et al.* BS. (1999). BCL-2 and p53 expression in clinically localized prostate cancer predicts response to external beam radiotherapy [published erratum appears in *J Urol* 1999; **162**: 503]. *Journal of Urology* **162**, 1–16

Schroder FH, Kranse R, Rietbergen J, Hoedemaeke R, Kirkels W (1999). The European Randomized Study of Screening for Prostate Cancer (ERSPC): an update. *European Urology* **35**, 539–543

Silberman MA, Partin AW, Veltri RW, Epstein JI (1997). Tumor angiogenesis correlates with progression after radical prostatectomy but not with pathologic stage in Gleason sum 5 to 7 adenocarcinoma of the prostate. *Cancer* **79**, 772–779

Stamey TA, Yang N, Hay AR, McNeal JE, Freiha FS, Redwine E (1987). Prostate-specific antigen as a serum marker for adenocarcinoma of the prostate. *New England Journal of Medicine* **317**, 909–916

Stamey TA, Kabalin JN, McNeal JE *et al.* (1989). Prostate specific antigen in the diagnosis and treatment of adenocarcinoma of the prostate. II. Radical prostatectomy treated patients. *Journal of Urology* **141**, 1076–1083

Ukimura O, Durrani O, Babaian RJ (1997). Role of PSA and its indices in determining the need for repeat prostate biopsies. *Urology* **50**, 66–72

Veltri RW, O'Dowd GJ, Orozco R, Miller MC (1998). The role of biopsy pathology, quantitative nuclear morphometry, and biomarkers in the preoperative prediction of prostate cancer staging and prognosis. *Seminars in Urology and Oncology* **16**, 106–117

Walsh PC (1998). Anatomic radical prostatectomy: evolution of the surgical technique. *Journal of Urology* **160**, 2418–2424

Walsh PC (2000). Radical prostatectomy for localized prostate cancer provides durable cancer control with excellent quality of life: a structured debate. *Journal of Urology* **163**, 1802–1807

Walsh PC, Partin AW, Epstein JI (1994). Cancer control and quality of life following anatomical radical retropubic prostatectomy: results at 10 years. *Journal of Urology* **152**, 1831–1836

Whitmore WF (1973). The natural history of prostatic cancer. *Cancer* **32**, 1104–1112

Wilson JMG & Jungner G (1969). *Principles and Practice of Screening for Disease.* Geneva: WHO, pp 1–34

Zincke H, Oesterling JE, Blute ML, Bergstralh EJ, Myers RP, Barrett DM (1994). Long-term (15 years) results after radical prostatectomy for clinically localized (stage T2c or lower) prostate cancer. *Journal of Urology* **152**, 1850–1857

Central determinants of clinical outcome: accelerating the clinical pathway from early diagnosis to institution of treatment

Hugh S Rogers

Introduction

Care of patients with cancer in Britain is not always good. It was recognised in 1999 that there was a clear need to improve care for patients with cancer. Delays were running at unacceptable levels, the patient journey was usually not very well co-ordinated and the public perception was that the service was poor. Work with redesign methods in the NHS, such as Leicester Royal Infirmary's re-engineering programme, the National Booked Admissions Programme (Meredith *et al.* 2000) and elsewhere (Berwick 1996, 1998; Berwick & Nolan 1998) had shown that improvement methodology could deliver major gains for patients without necessarily incurring unrealistic or prohibitive costs to the service.

The Cancer Services Collaborative project was set up to exploit these improvement methods and explore their ability to transform the treatment of patients with cancer in the NHS. The project ran from September 1999 until March 2001. Its aim was to improve the experience and outcomes for patients with suspected or diagnosed cancer. Nine sites across England worked on five cancers: prostate, breast, colorectal, lung and ovarian. Changes are made, initially on a small scale, in experimental cycles ('plan – do – study – act') (Moen *et al.* 1998).

Substantial changes have been made to the patient's pathway:

- Telephone booking, 'faxback' procedures and electronic referral protocols now allow the first specialist appointment to be given to patients before they leave the GP surgery.
- Time from referral to identification of patients at risk from prostate cancer has been reduced from 6 months to 10 days by a new nurse-led clinic.
- Pre-planning and booking a series of appointments for investigations and outpatient visits has reduced the maximum interval from a GP referring a patient 'at risk' of prostate cancer to the patient starting definitive treatment (such as radiotherapy or radical prostatectomy) from 35 weeks to just 7 weeks.
- Multidisciplinary patient records and logs of patient-held results have been developed.
- Patient information leaflets are now tailored to events along the patient journey.

Through the project, we have found ways to share new ideas and discovered the importance of clinicians in leading change. We have learned the power of process mapping and the impact of pre-booking, co-ordinating and simplifying the patient journey. We have reduced delays, improved access to care and increased patient satisfaction.

The problem

Waits and delays

Astonishing delays occur in cancer care in England (Spurgeon *et al.* 2000) and evidence is mounting to show that the delay from GP's referral to definitive treatment explains why cancer survival rates in the UK (Coleman *et al.* 1999) are lower than in the rest of Europe (Berrino *et al.* 1999). For suspected prostate cancer the average delay from urgent referral to first outpatient appointment was 3 weeks but two-thirds of patients with a final diagnosis of prostate cancer are referred non-urgently, mostly with lower urinary tract symptoms. These patients are seen and diagnosed much more slowly, from 13 weeks up to 6 months. Even when the patient has been seen in the hospital substantial delays may occur in carrying out investigations and reaching a diagnosis before treatment can be planned. Further delays can then occur before definitive treatment such as radiotherapy or radical surgery takes place (Table 4.1).

Table 4.1 Waiting times for prostate cancer patients in England (Spurgeon *et al.* 2000)

		Urgent referrals	Non-urgent referrals
Time to first outpatient appointment (days)	Median (interquartile range)	19 (9–29)	41 (23–56)
	When 90% of patients seen	44	77
Time to first definitive treatment (days)	Median (interquartile range)	53 (26–91)	111 (64–183)
	When 90% of patients treated	143	292

Poor co-ordination

Most cancer patients will say that they are satisfied with their care and grateful to the healthcare professionals whom they have encountered, but they are very unhappy with the way the system works and the delays that they incur along their journey. It is unusual to find any individual in an organisation who has an overview of the whole patient journey. The true complexity of that journey may be discovered only by walking through the process with a real patient. We find that the patient has little control over the process. There is usually no real choice about when their first appointment will be and little certainty about what will happen thereafter. Typically the cancer patient's journey is characterised by delays at each stage, patients having a series of visits for blood tests, radiographs, clinic consultations and so forth. There is poor co-ordination between different agencies and often it is left to the patient to make each appointment along the way. These difficulties are exaggerated when the care pathway involves more than one hospital.

Demand for better information

Patients now demand clear accessible information about their care and their condition. Excellent patient information exists in some units, but it tends to be patchy and often has little direct bearing on the needs of an individual patient at a crucial time in their life. Patients often seek further information from a variety of sources, e.g. patient helplines or support associations and the internet, but this information can be of variable quality, especially on the internet, and much of it is too broad and will not be directly relevant to that individual at that point in time.

Outline of the Cancer Services Collaborative Project

The Cancer Services Collaborative Project is transforming the care of patients with suspected or diagnosed cancer. This national project is funded by the NHS through the National Patients' Access Team. Phase 1 was funded for 18 months from September 1999 until March 2001. Programmes in nine separate cancer networks across England worked on five major cancers: prostate, breast, lung, colorectal and ovary. Eight of the nine networks ran prostate projects (Table 4.2).

Table 4.2 Geographical distribution of programmes

The Cancer Services Collaborative Project has projects in nine cancer networks:

Mid-Anglia Cancer Network (Eastern Region)
South East London Cancer Network (London Region)
West London Cancer Network (London Region)
Merseyside and Cheshire Cancer Zone (North West Region)
Northern Cancer Network (Northern and Yorkshire Region)[a]
Kent Cancer Network (South East Region)
Avon, Somerset and Wiltshire Cancer Services (South West Region)
Leicestershire Cancer Centre (Trent Region)
Birmingham Hospitals Cancer Network (West Midlands Region)

[a]Prostate projects were carried out in all except Northern Cancer Network.

The overall goal of the programme is to reduce delays and to redesign the system of delivering care in order to *improve the experience and outcomes for patients with suspected or diagnosed cancer*. Its purpose is to make the diagnosis rapidly and start treatment quickly and efficiently with care that is designed to suit the patient's needs, rather than the needs of the organisation that provides care. Its function is not to decide the most appropriate treatment for a particular cancer, although supporting clinical effectiveness in treatment is one of its aims. Don Berwick, Director of the Institute of Healthcare Improvement (IHI), has said 'Every system is perfectly designed to deliver precisely the results it achieves', a thought-provoking statement, the corollary to which is that if we do not like the results we have to change the system. Another way to express this is: 'If you always do what you've always done, you'll always get what you always got.' The improvement methodology developed by the IHI has been adopted within the Cancer Services Collaborative Project (Berwick 1998).[JS1]

Improvement methodology

This methodology has been adapted from that used by the IHI as described in the 'Breakthrough series' (Berwick & Nolan 1998; Clemmer 1998; Nelson 1998; Reinerstein 1998). The model is based on scientific method and is intended to develop a culture of continuing improvement. It is based on three fundamental questions:

- What are we trying to accomplish? (Aims)
- How will we know if a change is an improvement? (Measures)
- What changes can we make that will result in improvement? (Redesign)

The method is based on the experimental principle of making a change and observing the result. The experiments begin on a small scale to reduce risk and help to allay the resistance of sceptics. The incremental approach also makes it possible to approach a large and complex process such as the cancer patient journey (Figure 4.1) in manageable elements.

Staff teams meet regularly with the project manager to consider progress made and come up with suggestions for improvement. Ideas come from the administrative and clerical staff as often as from the clinical staff on the team (nursing, medical, etc.). Any idea of how we could do something better is tried out on a small scale to find out whether it works and what repercussions it may have. The outcomes of this small change cycle are reviewed. If successful, the idea is modified as necessary and tested again on a larger sample. In practice, this may mean trying a new idea on a single patient, then a single clinic session, before implementing it more widely, gradually building up the experience to the whole service or discarding it. We learn more from what does not work than from what does work because, if an idea is shown not to work, it need not be explored further. A successful new process may have alternatives, which may be just as successful or more so.

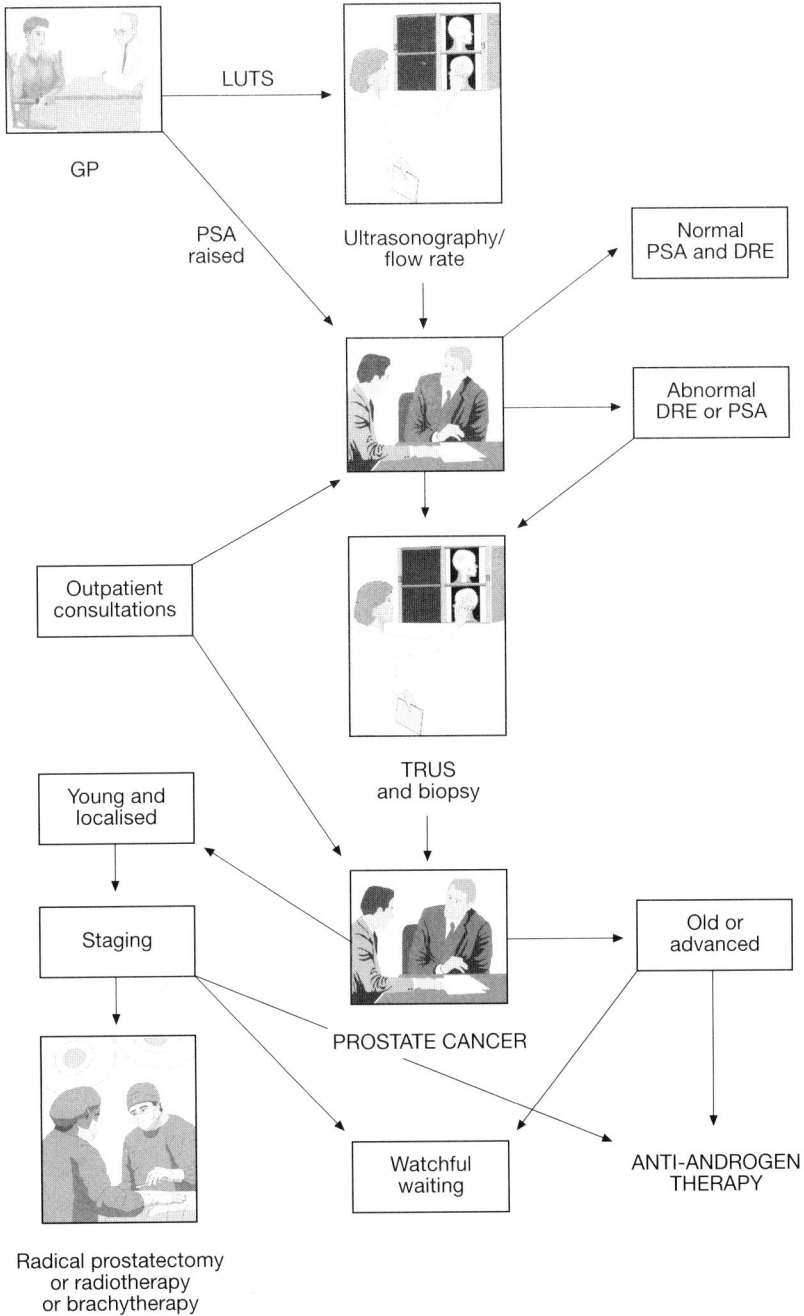

Figure 4.1 The complexity of the patient pathway for prostate cancer. GP, general practitioner; LUTS, lower urinary tract symptoms; PSA, prostate-specific antigen; DRE, digital rectal examination; TRUS, transrectal ultrasonography.

Aims of the project

At the start each of the 43 project teams created a set of aims statements consistent with the goals of the collaborative. We set ourselves challenging targets at the outset (Table 4.3), but modified some of these and have added to them over time as the relative importance of different targets became apparent. Aims must include aspects that can be measured in some way. Targets are set and graphs or 'run charts' of these measures are plotted over time to demonstrate progress towards the targets. The run charts can demonstrate the impact of changes at given points in time (Figure 4.2).

Table 4.3 Aims at the start of the project (some of these were modified later in the light of experience)

	Aim	Measure
Access	100% of referrals seen within national waiting times but strive to continuous improvement throughout project	Proportion of patients seen within national waiting times
Access (sub-aims)[a]	100% of urgent referrals seen within 2 weeks	Proportion of patients seen within target times
	80% of all other referrals seen within 28 days	
	100% commence first definitive treatment within 3 weeks of diagnosis	
Patient flow	90% of patients booked in advance for the next stage in their journey	Proportion of total care process booked in advance
Information flow	90% of the appropriate information accessible at the appropriate time	Proportion of appropriate information accessible at any key stage in the patient journey
Patient satisfaction	90% of patients give score of 4 or 5 on a 5-point scale for whole patient journey	Satisfaction scores for whole journey on a 5-point scale
Clinical effectiveness	95% of patients managed in accordance with current best practice	Percentage managed in accordance with current best practice
Capacity and demand	For all of key stages demand assessed and capacity controlled	The proportion of patients who receive planned care within agreed waiting times across key stages of patient journey
	All patients seen within target times	

[a]All criteria had detailed 'sub-aims' but only those for access are shown.

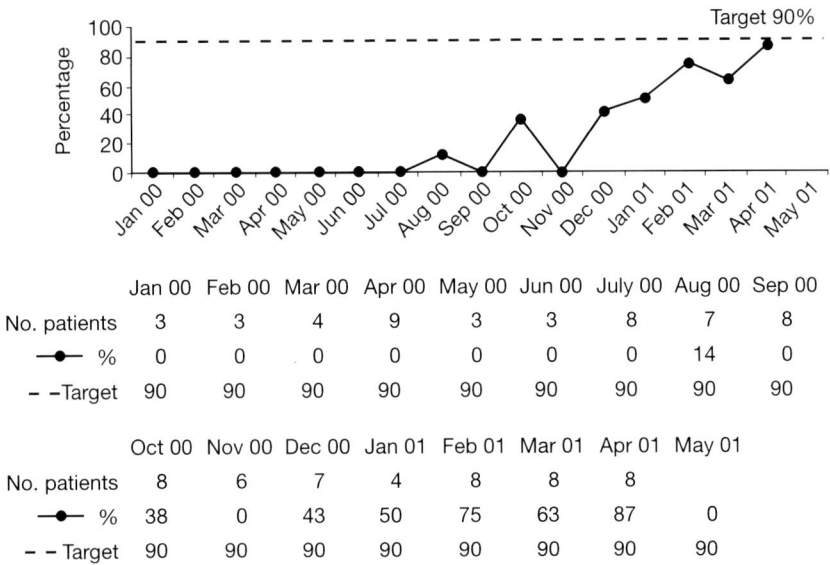

	Jan 00	Feb 00	Mar 00	Apr 00	May 00	Jun 00	July 00	Aug 00	Sep 00
No. patients	3	3	4	9	3	3	8	7	8
—●— %	0	0	0	0	0	0	0	14	0
– –Target	90	90	90	90	90	90	90	90	90

	Oct 00	Nov 00	Dec 00	Jan 01	Feb 01	Mar 01	Apr 01	May 01
No. patients	8	6	7	4	8	8	8	
—●— %	38	0	43	50	75	63	87	0
– – Target	90	90	90	90	90	90	90	90

Figure 4.2 Run chart to show the percentage of patients booked by their GP for first specialist appointment. The new faxback procedures were started in August, the first GPs were introduced to the system at that time, and the scheme was extended to further GPs by December. The aim was for all GPs to use the system by April and the target was that 90% of referrals should be booked.

We monitor time delays for each element of the patient journey and overall times from referral to diagnosis and to treatment (Figure 4.3). Patient satisfaction is assessed through a variety of tools such as questionnaires, focus groups and interviews. These explore the system of care and the information and support given through the journey. Some programmes are using similar tools to assess GP satisfaction.

Co-ordinating the patient journey

To co-ordinate the journey for suspected cancer patients, the Cancer Services Collaborative Project sets out to map the process from GP referral to diagnosis and treatment (Layton *et al.* 1998). We set out to transform the procedures for GP referral, principally by direct booking of the first appointment, and then to ensure that any sequence of consultations and investigations is planned and pre-scheduled right up to the decision on treatment. Once the treatment is agreed, surgical or otherwise, that too is pre-planned and booked in order to give the patient a clear plan of action and remove uncertainty.

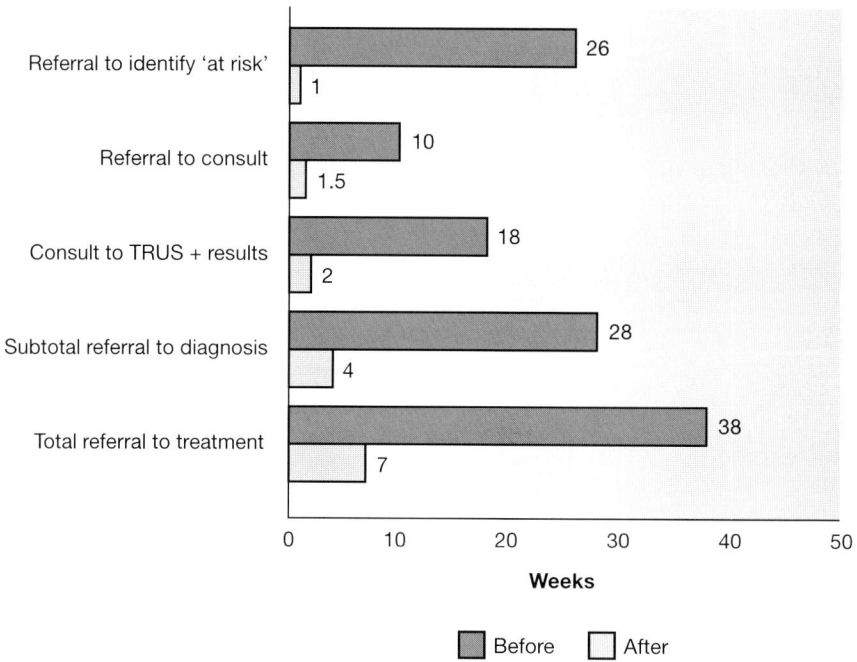

Figure 4.3 Transformed waiting times – maximum delays in weeks. TRUS, transrectal ultrasonography.

Improving the patient experience

To improve patients' experiences further we wanted to give them better understanding of the procedures at each stage. We canvassed patients' views and monitored patient satisfaction in order to find what patients need most. We wanted to increase patient control by booking the journey to allow care to be tailored to the individual. We developed information materials to correspond to patients' feedback.

Optimising delivery of care

New ways of organising and delivering care were tried by reorganising the way administrative and clerical staff support the patient journey. We explored the role of alternative providers of care for particular groups of patients, supported by protocols. Developments included extending the role of the nurse specialist in providing nurse-led outpatient clinics. The traditional view of 'routine' hospital follow-up was challenged and some services were relocated to improve the patient's journey.

Matching capacity and demand

Process mapping was used to identify bottle-necks and constraints in the system that required analysis to determine the best solutions. The work falls into four phases:

- analyse and predict true demand and patient need
- eliminate backlogs
- realise the true capacity
- manage capacity in order to match demand on a daily basis (anticipating and planning for changes in capacity as a result of holidays, etc.).

A common fallacy is to assume that a long waiting time represents a mismatch of capacity and demand, whereas a stable waiting time, however long, indicates that throughput and demand are equal. It is often assumed that clearing a backlog will increase demand, but for many procedures (such as histopathology) this is unlikely. Where it is true (e.g. in radiology) other methods can be used to manage demand, such as protocols for referral, or alternative paths can be evolved to relieve pressure at the constraint, such as nurse-led clinics for defined groups of patients to take pressure off consultant clinics.

The analogy of the water tank with water flowing in at the top and flowing out through the bottom illustrates the idea. Lowering the overall level (i.e. reducing delay by eliminating backlogs) does not necessarily have an impact on either the inflow (demand) or the outflow (capacity). However, short-term restrictions in capacity (e.g. holidays of key staff) can have a long-term impact on delays. They need to be predicted and allowance made for them by planning capacity to prevent this. Simply clearing a backlog is seldom the whole answer because, unless the issue of matching capacity to demand is addressed as well, the waiting time will usually return to its previous level as anyone associated with waiting list initiatives in the NHS will confirm. ('If you don't like the results you have to change the system.')

One way of dealing with bottle-necks is to find some patients who can follow an alternative pathway (see Example 7). Sometimes the only answer is to increase capacity by increasing resources, but analysis can show whether the need is for extra equipment or for more staff and an innovative approach can direct investment into the most appropriate staff (Goldratt 1993).

Experiences during the Cancer Collaborative Project

Early findings

Many projects found examples of excellent practices already in existence, but only in a few cases did good practice extend across the whole process from referral to treatment. Some departments were booking urgent patients using a variety of methods, but most did not allow for patient choice in this process. A few were pre-scheduling more than one visit (e.g. ultrasonography before consultation), but this tended to be patchy and usually only covered one or two steps in the pathway.

There were (and still are in places) delays and bottle-necks in the patient journey. The most important bottle-necks we found were at initial consultation, at diagnostic tests such as transrectal ultrasonography and bone scans, and at radiotherapy.

Long delays have been found in histopathology, which seem hard to understand because the processing of samples usually takes just a few hours. Most of the delay is spent waiting between various different stages of the process. Redesign in these circumstances can have a dramatic impact; in one unit turn-round times have been cut from 3 weeks to 3 hours.

Small-scale testing

Testing on a small scale has proved to have many advantages. Unsuccessful ideas are discarded before any damage is done. Radical changes can be introduced gradually without great upheaval, and the incremental approach helps to overcome resistance to change by showing evidence of tangible benefits. This approach has been used throughout the cancer collaborative to introduce change in a non-threatening way, but it has led to radical improvement of whole systems in many parts of the patient journey.

Process mapping

The process is mapped out by all key participants in the patient pathway coming together and charting in detail the overall patient journey for the typical patient. This meeting is key to understanding and agreeing the true process, and it yields many surprises for members of the team who come to appreciate the whole journey for the first time (Layton *et al.* 1998). Mapping the process in detail has proved to be a very powerful tool in revealing why the system needs to be simplified, and it starts to identify some obvious bottle-necks and delays.

Sometimes, when considered in isolation, each step of a process seems acceptable. A wait of up to 2 weeks for a first consultation may seem reasonable. Two weeks for transrectal ultrasonography (TRUS) and prostate biopsy, and a further 2 weeks to see the urologist may seem acceptable. Then, after sending a referral letter, a wait of 2 weeks to see the radiotherapist and another 2 weeks before the start of treatment seems reasonable, yet, when the steps in the journey are added together, the delay from referral to treatment is 10 weeks. In practice we have found that the delays in some of these steps can be much longer.

Most people worrying about the prospect of cancer would find such delays unacceptable, so much so that it is common practice for staff working in the health service to use personal contacts to find ways of accelerating the pathway for themselves and their families. How then can such delays be acceptable for the population we serve?

Capacity and demand

Measuring true demand and matching it to real capacity have been important tools in dealing with bottle-necks in the system.

Example 1

> The breast clinic at West Middlesex had a long backlog for non-urgent mammography. Up to half the patients with cancer came from the non-urgent group, so we determined that we would treat all patients with breast lumps rapidly. Analysis showed that there were too few non-urgent slots to meet demand, but too many slots had been reserved for the urgent patients. By redressing the balance, and by planning sessions to allow for holidays, capacity equalled demand. The backlog was eliminated by validating the list and providing extra sessions. Now all patients have their mammogram on the day of their first appointment.

The conclusions of analysis are often counter-intuitive. Delays in radiology are common and most people assume that to solve this more machines are needed. Analysis often demonstrates that the existing machines are not being used efficiently. Accurately matching booked slots to the time taken for the procedure, reducing wasted slots resulting from cancellations or from patients who do not attend (see Example 3) and encouraging staff to work more flexibly can realise substantial increases in capacity. The solution to achieving this may be extra clinical staff time or increased clerical input but process redesign may reduce downtime and increase throughput without any extra resources.

Example 2

> The South East London prostate project found long delays for bone scans. Patients were booked for 30-min slots but, although larger patients took 30 min, short slim patients took much less time. The referring doctor now communicates the size of the patient on the request form, allowing appropriate time to be booked on the scanner. This has increased capacity sufficiently to eliminate the backlog completely.

Redesign and innovation

Involving patients in booking their appointments rather than sending appointments to them has already been shown dramatically to reduce the number of patients who cancel appointments or fail to attend in our hospital.

Example 3

> At West Middlesex, moving from a conventional waiting list to a system in which the patient books their appointment for day surgery procedures has given patients more control and increased their commitment to the booked date. As a result the incidence of patient-initiated cancellations has fallen from 5% to 2% and the number who fail to attend on the day of surgery ('DNAs') has fallen from 7.7% to 1.2%, with consequent increases in efficiency for the hospital.

Onward referrals from secondary to tertiary care traditionally happen by formal letter. The doctor dictates a letter and passes the tape to the secretary who types it and sends it in the post. The mailroom staff sort it and deliver it, the receiving secretary opens it and passes it to her consultant for review of priority. Finally a clinic clerk sends an appointment to the patient by post. At least six people are involved, each of whom may think that they are doing their job well, but the number of different steps in the process mounts up. The whole process may take several weeks before the patient attends their appointment to plan treatment. Using a fax machine can shorten the process somewhat, but a more radical view can achieve even greater overall gains.

Example 4

> After discussion with consultants at the tertiary centre, patients needing radical radiotherapy are booked by telephone from the urology clinic at the secondary unit directly into a radiotherapy planning session, and those requiring radical surgery are booked directly into the relevant surgeon's clinic. The patients are seen in less than one week, and in the case of radiotherapy treatment starts at once. The surgeon plans a provisional date for surgery on receipt of the referral before seeing the patient.

Patient involvement

Patients' views have been canvassed in a number of ways. Questionnaires can be useful to assess particular issues, such as patient information leaflets. Patient support groups have also helped us to redesign information leaflets around the questions that they are frequently asked. We have convened groups of patients who have been through the process, and discussed their experiences and suggestions for improvement of the system. All these methods have their drawbacks. Questionnaires are a crude way of evaluating the patient experience and have limited value in assessing patient satisfaction. Support groups may not reflect the diversity of patient experience and tend to focus on the bigger picture rather than details of the process. Focus groups may be useful but impractical for groups of patients who may be sick, such as groups of lung cancer patients.

The most powerful and open-ended way to discover the real patient experience is to accompany a patient on visits to find out what actually happens along the journey and how the patient reacts. This can reveal important insights about failings in the system and gives the most dramatic insights into the patient's experience.

Reorganising the service around the patient

At West Middlesex we have found that having a single team responsible for the whole patient journey has led to better co-ordination of the urology department and the patient processes in it. In the old system, the outpatient staff were separated managerially and physically from the urology department secretaries. We merged the teams, and put them together in an integrated urology unit. The staff are now able to cover each others' roles and we all work as a team. Instead of blaming each other (e.g. 'we don't have the notes as the secretaries have got them' or 'the clinic staff have lost the results'), we work together and take joint responsibility for sorting out any problems. All members of the team have direct access to the medical and nursing staff in the unit to resolve queries. In the event of sickness or holidays, they cover for each other because all can do reception duty and all understand the office procedures.

Dictated letters have almost become obsolete because the outcome of clinic consultations is recorded on a standard proforma. This is faxed or sent by post to the GP at the end of the clinic and a copy made for the notes. Onward referrals to tertiary care are made by faxing a similar standard proforma letter after the appointment has been booked by telephone.

We are piloting on-screen entry of clinic outcomes into a standard template. This opens up the potential to transmit the clinic outcome letter electronically into the GP's system or into another hospital.

Many unnecessary follow-ups have been prevented by a 'paper clinic' at which the notes and results are reviewed in the absence of the patient. The outcome of this is communicated to the patient and GP.

Example 5

Histology of prostate biopsies is reviewed in the 'paper clinic'. Those patients with benign biopsies are telephoned to give them the good news. If no follow-up is felt necessary the patient's appointment is cancelled to leave more time for those whose biopsies show cancer. Similarly we review the histology of all patients having transurethral resection of the prostate (TURP). Those with cancer on histology are recalled for follow-up, but there is an open door policy to allow any others with problems to return easily if they wish.

The key changes to achieve improvements

During the programme the eight project teams have tested thousands of ideas. We have now developed a consensus about those changes that have the most impact in improving the system.

Booking the appointment reduces delay and cuts DNAs

At the start of the project, new procedures were already being introduced by most trusts to comply with the national standard to see all 'suspected cancer' referrals within 2 weeks ('2-week wait guidelines'). This accelerated the change process because there is an obligation to see all patients marked by the GP as 'suspected cancer' within 2 weeks of referral. It thereby removed the need to prioritise those referrals and simplified the process. We have found that booking first appointments has been of additional value in bypassing slow and bureaucratic referral mechanisms and giving patients some influence over their appointments.

We have tested a variety of new ways to book urgent patients from GP to first appointment:

- Tumour-specific paper fax proformas have proved not to be acceptable to GPs. At the introduction of the '2-week wait standards' for urgent breast referrals such proformas seemed to be successful, but GPs are now being asked to take on an increasing number of proformas, which they refuse to use. The reason given for this is that they only refer an urgent 'suspected cancer' patient once a week or less and GPs do not have systems in place to deal with a variety of different proformas that are seldom used. We are now testing a generic proforma across the local cancer network with the '2-week wait' criteria printed on the cover for reference.
- Telephone booking has the advantage that it gives patients an opportunity to agree an appointment that suits them. It gives them choice and control while reducing cancellations and failures to attend. However, it is labour intensive.
- An innovation called the 'Faxback' procedure has been successfully piloted. The GP's receptionist sends a letter or proforma by fax to the clinic and is immediately sent a response with the date, time and place of the appointment, with any supporting information necessary. The patient leaves the GP surgery with the appointment and whatever other information the hospital chooses to send. If patients find that the appointment is difficult for them and they wish to change it, a telephone number is given for them to ring. This has been so successful in creating confidence in both the GP and the patient that this procedure is now being extended to all referrals for 'suspected cancer' in the hospital, using a single central fax line. The only disadvantage is that the process does not allow true choice for the patient who must call in by telephone if the appointment offered does not suit them.
- We are currently testing interactive electronic booking procedures in which the GP links to our systems over the NHS Net. They have to navigate a short clinical protocol but, provided the referral meets the criteria, they can book the appointment themselves. Electronic direct booking gives certainty to patients and GPs and allows patients to choose a suitable appointment. The other solutions above are probably interim solutions. We are convinced that this method of referral will supersede all others, provided that sufficient lessons are learned to allow GPs to accept it as the normal way for them to transfer care.

Pre-scheduling and pre-planning

Pre-scheduling a series of visits for appointments, investigations and results is a good way to give greater certainty to the patient while substantially reducing delays.

Example 6

> In West London patients referred by their GP with a raised prostate-specific antigen (PSA) test have a series of visits booked from the outset. They are seen in a urology clinic within 7 days of referral to review the need for biopsy, which is then carried out within 4 days. The visit for results is booked 3 days later on the day of the multidisciplinary team meeting, so the diagnosis is made within 14 days of the GP referral. This is half the time given in the cancer plan targets (NHS Cancer Plan 2000). All three visits are planned from the outset and the multidisciplinary meeting is scheduled. Other projects have gone one step further and carry out the biopsy on the same day as the initial consultation.

Matching capacity and demand

Bottle-necks at the new patient appointment stage are relieved by reducing unnecessary follow-ups (see Example 9) and by diverting patients to alternative pathways.

Example 7

> Formerly, patients referred with lower urinary tract symptoms (LUTS) were sent for ultrasonography and routine blood tests before their first appointment. The letter was prioritised and an ultrasonography request generated (2 weeks). The patient waited for the ultrasonography appointment (14 weeks) and had their blood tests at the same visit. Then they had to book their consultation (10 weeks later). The total delay before recognising that a patient may be 'at risk' of having prostate cancer on the basis of a raised PSA level was 6 months. A new nurse-led clinic was set up in which patients with LUTS are seen within 7 days of referral. They are assessed using a protocol, their blood tests are taken and they undergo ultrasonography in the urology department. At review the following week with results of the PSA, all the 'at-risk' patients in this group are identified within 14 days of referral. These patients are discussed with a urologist and booked for a TRUS and biopsy within 5 days.

The demand for TRUS and biopsy is relatively small compared with the overall workload in radiology. Nevertheless, it has taken almost 12 months to improve the service in order to eliminate the backlog and book patients directly.

Example 8

> Only two transrectal ultrasonographic examinations of the prostate with biopsy (TRUS and biopsy) were carried out every 2 weeks in a satellite hospital where the radiologist felt confident in the nursing care. The urology department was on the main site, so dislocation of the service impaired any attempt at service redesign and many patients were unhappy travelling to the less accessible site. After several unsuccessful attempts to move the service, the project manager, a nurse, suggested that a single patient should have the procedure at the main hospital. She arranged the equipment, booked and counselled the patient, and came to support the radiologist during and after the procedure. After larger trials, new biopsy equipment was bought at minimal cost and the radiology

department now supports the service in the new location. The consultant radiologist has recognised the advantages to patients of moving the service and the capacity has been increased to three slots weekly.

Follow-up

Several projects have reviewed the value of 'routine' follow-up for the five tumours in the programme. Evidence shows that it may have no clinical benefit for some tumours because patients with relapsing disease notice new symptoms themselves and very few are discovered unexpectedly at the time of clinic review. In the case of prostate cancer, stable disease is monitored by regular PSA blood tests. Some urologists have transferred stable patients to their GP colleagues for regular review; others have set up nurse specialist follow-up clinics. In every case there are two prerequisites for transferring follow-up to alternative providers of care:

1. Patients need education about the limited benefits of follow-up and the sort of symptoms they should regard as potentially sinister.
2. Direct access must be provided for patients to return to the clinic promptly if they develop any worrying symptoms.

Patients need a direct telephone line to obtain advice if they have any concerns. This is usually best provided by a competent nurse specialist who is qualified to provide advice and can judge the need for review either by herself or in the medical clinic.

Example 9

Audit of patients undergoing follow-up after treatment of breast cancer at Mount Vernon Hospital showed that in 5 years on average they had 13 visits and were seen by nine different doctors. A focus group of patients was brought together to discuss follow-up. Once they understood the limited benefit of follow-up (other than routine mammography), they were asked what form of follow-up they would prefer. Offered the choice of GP or specialist nurse follow-up, they opted to have no routine follow-up at all provided that they could telephone the specialist nurse if they had any concerns.

Involvement of the specialist nurse

We have learned the pivotal role of the specialist nurse in urology. The nurse has a major role providing clinical care to patients whether doing nurse-led clinics (see Example 7), contributing to care of patients undergoing biopsies or supporting them through the time of diagnosis or relapse.

One of their most important roles is in educating and informing patients so as to help them to understand their condition and alternative options for treatment. They are well placed to co-ordinate the contributions of various departments and agencies to the complex supportive care of patients with advanced disease.

They usually stay in post much longer than junior doctors and become well known to the patients and GPs. By making themselves available by telephone, they offer security to patients who find it comforting to be able to turn to someone who knows them, who is familiar with their condition and treatment, and who can advise them about problems large and small.

Nurses have sometimes been strong advocates for change. The concept of building services round patient needs comes more naturally to nurses than to some doctors. Many of the successful project managers in the cancer collaborative programme have a nursing background.

Better information along the journey
Patient information

We encourage all patients to discuss their individual position and treatment options with the urology nurse specialist (and for advanced cases the palliative care nurses as well), but written information is a valuable adjunct. Patient feedback has taught us that most patients do not want comprehensive information booklets covering all aspects of their cancer. Most patients find too much information difficult to assimilate and to relate to their own position. If a patient is struggling over the implications of an abnormal PSA result, there is no point in trying to tell him everything about prostate cancer from A to Z because that is not usually what he wants at the time. We have found that patients prefer concise information leaflets specifically covering the implications of their own clinical condition and the procedures that they are to undergo at particular stages in the journey.

We have written several patient leaflets specific to different stages in the journey. In this task we have benefited from helpful contributions from patient support associations as well as current patients. Text has been shared between different projects (by email) and customised, adding local detail such as the contact numbers for the clinic receptionist and specialist nurse, and a map to show where the department is.

There will always be some patients who want a more detailed in-depth understanding. The nurse specialist can offer them alternative sources of reliable information, including reference books, patient support helplines and worthwhile internet sites.

Patient-held record

Prostate cancer lends itself particularly well to a patient-held record because PSA is such an accurate indicator of disease activity and response to treatment. We introduced a small booklet in which we record the date of diagnosis, the PSA level and the initial treatment. Thereafter, we record PSA levels and changes of treatment on each visit. This has the advantage that all healthcare professionals dealing with the patient can refer to the log as a concise record of the time course of treatment and activity of the disease. It has proved popular with patients (who, we discovered, frequently record their results anyway) but has the added benefits of reducing duplication of PSA testing and greatly improving communication between different clinics (e.g. urology clinic, radiotherapy unit, GP surgery). Other projects (e.g. breast project) have introduced hand-held multidisciplinary records covering the whole care pathway.

Impact of improvements on the patient's experience

Key achievements

- Protocol-based electronic booking commenced for GP referrals
- Creation of nurse-led lower urinary tract symptom and follow-up clinics
- Maximum wait for 'at-risk' patients to be identified from non-urgent referrals with lower urinary tract symptoms reduced from 26 weeks to 2 weeks
- Direct booking for first appointment, diagnostic test and results clinic
- Direct booking for radiotherapy and surgery to another hospital
- Re-location of TRUS and biopsies to the main hospital
- Maximum time from GP referral to definitive surgery reduced from 36 weeks to 7 weeks
- Patient-held record (PSA log book)
- New patient information leaflets devised
- Introduction of 'paper clinic'
- Joint oncology clinic established
- Reduced delays.

Within the programme we have agreed an ideal journey for prostate cancer with recommended maximum timescales (Figure 4.4). The agreed maximum time from referral to treatment was 9 weeks. This is slightly outside the 2005 national cancer plan target (two calendar months), so we need to reduce this further. In practice most projects have already exceeded this target including our own (see Figure 4.3). For most patients with prostate cancer the initial treatment is hormonal manipulation so this will normally be started in clinic at the time of diagnosis, within 3 weeks of the initial referral (Figure 4.4).

An important principle has been established. The system should set target times to complete the various stages but, if the patient chooses to delay, for whatever reason, we should try to meet the patient's needs. Such delays need recording to make it clear that we are fulfilling our own obligations, and analysis of the reasons patients give for delay will be interesting in due course to inform future work.

All the other tumour groups have agreed a maximum interval from referral to definitive treatment of less that 2 months and this work was used in setting the targets in the NHS Cancer Plan of 2 months for all cancers by 2005 (NHS Cancer Plan 2000).

```
                    ┌──────────────┐   1/52 →  ┌──────────────┐
                    │  GP refers   │──────────→│  Nurse-led   │
                    │   patient    │           │ 'LUTS' clinic│
                    └──────────────┘           └──────────────┘
                         │                         │
                      2/52                       1/52
                         ↓                         ↓
                    ┌──────────────┐
                    │ Urologist-led│
                    │   clinic +   │
                    │  TRUS/biopsy │
                    └──────────────┘
                         │
                      1/52
                         ↓
                    ┌──────────────┐           ┌──────────────┐
                    │   Results    │─────────→ │  Majority:   │
                    │    clinic    │           │  hormonal    │
                    └──────────────┘           │ manipulation │
                         │                     └──────────────┘
                      2/52                     ┌──────────────────┐
                         ↓                     │ Total 3/52 – 5/52│
                    ┌──────────────┐           └──────────────────┘
                    │  MDT clinic  │
                    │Treatment plan│
                    └──────────────┘
                         │
                      4/52
                         ↓
                    ┌──────────────┐
                    │   Radical    │
                    │  treatment   │
                    └──────────────┘
                    ┌──────────────┐
                    │  Total 9/52  │
                    └──────────────┘
```

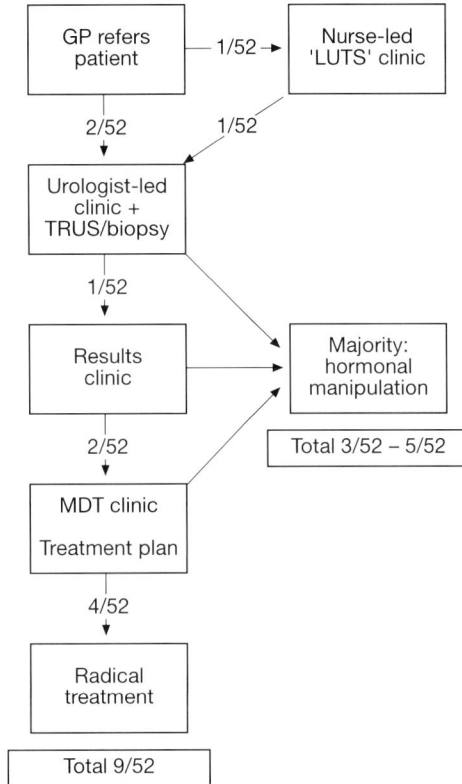

Figure 4.4 The ideal journey for prostate cancer.

Benefits to patients

In addition to dramatic reductions in delays we have demonstrated substantial tangible improvements for patients. Pre-scheduling and co-ordinating the journey are much appreciated by patients because it improves certainty about the process and confidence in the system. Booking adds a measure of control for the patient. Patients tell us that they are well informed and supported through the journey. Patient satisfaction levels measured on a five-point scale have risen substantially through the life of the project.

Learning from the project

During phase 1 of the Cancer Services Collaborative many new lessons have been learned:

- A trained project manager with strong facilitation skills is important to ensure that all members of the team can make their contribution, to implement the agreed changes and to measure the impact of change.

- The use of small change cycles works well in the NHS culture. It overcomes resistance to change and develops ownership of new processes by the team who develop them. This means that they have a stake in sustaining the new processes.
- The importance of clinical leadership has emerged as a critical factor in creating sustainable change. During the project several natural leaders have emerged from the clinicians in the programme, many of whom were highly sceptical at first.
- At the beginning of the project there was widespread resistance to change from both clinical staff and others. This can be characterised as the 'not invented here' syndrome and often expressed as: 'you don't understand, it wouldn't work here' or 'I've got a good way of doing that already, I don't need to change'. The converse of this was a reluctance to share good ideas. This arises from a spirit of competition which was fostered by the development of the internal market in health care and particularly the desire of hospitals to attract more referrals from GP fund-holding practices. At first it was hard to convince colleagues that we should share good ideas to the benefit of all our patients. In practice the competitive spirit has now been turned to the advantage of the project because different project groups have struggled to outdo each other in innovations and measured improvements, yet have learned the mutual benefit of sharing ideas. We have coined the phrase 'noble plagiarism' and have given awards for it. We have learned better ways to share ideas and adopted the slogan 'all teach all learn'. Written information is best disseminated by electronic file transfer so that it can be edited or customised for local use. Achieving consensus on ideal pathways, innovation in redesign and ways to optimise procedures have been successfully shared between projects at residential workshops where cross-fertilisation of ideas may happen equally in the conference room and the bar.

Dissemination of innovation

The NHS Cancer Plan sets ambitious targets for waiting times. By 2005 we must reduce the interval from GP referral to first definitive treatment down to 2 months for all cancers. The redesign methods of the Cancer Services Collaborative will be one of the key strategies to move towards these targets, along with investment in staff and equipment. The redesign methods, and particularly the work on matching capacity and demand, will help to identify those elements of the service where such investment will be most beneficial.

National output from phase 1 of the programme has been published as Service Improvement Guides (2001). These guides report a variety of ways in which projects have approached common problems and solved them in their local context. They do not claim to be prescriptive and recognise that different environments may require different local solutions. They give descriptions of ideas, approaches or innovations that have worked and may be worth trying, with contact details of the key individuals involved in the change.

Phase 2 of the Cancer Services Collaborative Project is to run for 2 years from April 2001 and involves every cancer network. The objectives of phase 2 are to spread the learning in the existing five cancers to new networks and new hospitals while simultaneously applying the improvement approach to new anatomical sites: upper gastrointestinal cancers, all urological and all gynaecological cancers. Research on how new ideas are adopted shows that, once a critical mass of about 20% is achieved, a change or innovation may become self-perpetuating (Rogers 1995). Provided that this critical mass can be achieved in phase 2 of the programme, mechanisms to enable further spread to occur are in place:

The cancer networks will increasingly be responsible for delivering the cancer plan targets so they will work to spread good practice within their network. They have the advantage that they are already working across established clinical networks. They have set up tumour boards for the major cancers so they have structures through which to disseminate new ways of working.

The National 'Booked Admission' project is funded to continue until at least 2003. This has gone well beyond its original remit and will support the booking of all parts of a patient journey. One of the priorities for the fourth wave of the 'booked admissions' project is to roll out booking of the cancer patient's journey during 2001–2003.

Professional bodies could have an important role in disseminating new ideas. Their endorsement can be a powerful way of communicating the improvement methodology. In some cases this has happened but some professional associations have been slow to rise to the challenge.

Conclusion

The Cancer Services Collaborative Project has succeeded in using improvement methodology to transform the experience for patients with suspected or diagnosed cancer within the programme. The interval from referral to treatment has been dramatically reduced by a variety of innovations. The most effective changes have been:

- booking the initial consultation
- redesigning and pre-planning the subsequent sequence of visits through diagnosis and treatment
- matching capacity and demand
- realising the importance of the specialist nurse and of targeted information.

Lessons have been learned about introducing innovation and how to share good practice. The redesign methodology of the Cancer Services Collaborative Project is now the key strategy to achieve the ambitious targets of the National Cancer Plan and the central role of clinical leaders has been recognised in the spread programme of phase 2. The challenge now is to ensure diffusion of the cultural change throughout the NHS, so that continuous development of services based on improving the patient's experience becomes a core element of the management of all clinical services.

References

Berwick D (1996). A primer on leading the improvement of systems. *British Medical Journal* **312**, 619–622

Berwick D (1998). Developing and testing changes in delivery of care. *Annals of Internal Medicine* **128**, 651–658

Berwick D & Nolan T (1998). Physicians as leaders in improving health care: a new series in annals of internal medicine. *Annals of Internal Medicine* **128**, 289–292

Berrino F *et al.* (1999). *Survival of Cancer Patients in Europe: the EUROCARE study II*. IARC Scientific Publication No 151. Lyon: IARC

Clemmer P *et al.* (1998). Cooperation: the foundations of improvement. *Annals of Internal Medicine* **128**, 1004–1009

Coleman M *et al.* (1999). *Cancer Survival Trends in England and Wales 1971–1995: Deprivation and NHS region*. London: The Stationery Office

Goldratt E (1993). *The Goal,* 2nd edn. Aldershot: Gower Publishing

Layton A, Moss F, Morgan G (1998). Mapping out the patient's journey: experiences of developing pathways of care. *Quality in Health Care* **7**(suppl), S30–S36

Meredith P, Ham C, Kipping R (2000). Modernising the NHS: Booking patients for hospital care. First interim report from the evaluation of the National Booked Admissions Programme: www.doh.gov.uk/bookedadmissions

Moen R, Nolan T, Provost L (1998). *Quality Improvement through Planned Experimentation,* 2nd edn. New York: McGraw Hill

Murray M (2000). Modernising the NHS – patient care: access. *British Medical Journal* **320**, 1594–1596

Nelson E *et al.* (1998). Building measurement and data collection into medical practice. *Annals of Internal Medicine* **128**, 460–466

NHS Cancer Plan (2000). Department of Health: www.doh.gov.uk/cancer

Reinerstein J (1998). Physicians as leaders in the improvement of health care systems. *Annals of Internal Medicine* **128**, 833–838

Rogers EM (1995). *Diffusion of Innovations*, 4th edn. New York: The Free Press, Simon & Schuster

Service Improvement Guides (2001). National Patient Access Team, 4th Floor St John's House, East Street, Leicester: www.nhs.uk/npat

Spurgeon P, Barwell F, Kerr D (2000) Waiting times for cancer patients in England after general practitioners' referrals: retrospective national survey. *British Medical Journal* **320**, 838–839

PART 3

Evidence and opinion for clinical intervention

The scientific evidence and expert opinion based on surgical intervention in prostate cancer

Amir V Kaisary, Ross Knight and Michael Jarmulowicz

Introduction

Prostate cancer has been overshadowed in the past by other cancers in men, namely lung and colon cancer. However, over the last few years, increased awareness has made it move up the scale and it is now acknowledged as possibly the second killer disease in men. It is acceptable that there are variations between races and countries, which would dictate the relative value of the disease in each particular country.

The life expectancy data and expectations in UK men (1911–2021) are shown in Figure 5.1 (Office for National Statistics 2000). It is of vital importance to men diagnosed in their early 40s to address the question of prostatic carcinoma with regard to treatment. Epidemiological studies have identified high-grade prostatic intraepithelial neoplasia (PIN) as a valuable finding in biopsy specimens which

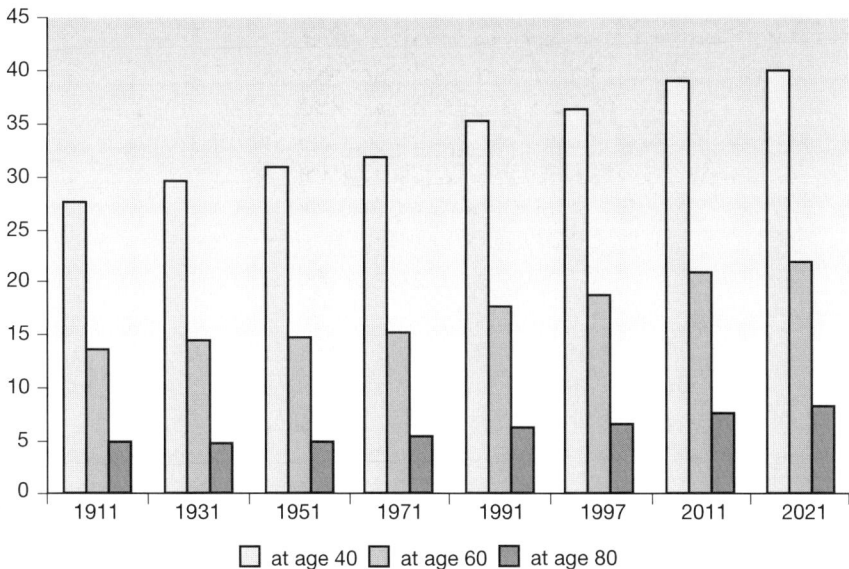

Figure 5.1 Expectation of life in UK men (1911–2021).

would warrant careful evaluation because, if left untreated, it would progress to adenocarcinoma (Bostwick 1999). The current approach of clinical evaluation and investigations include digital rectal examination (DRE), prostatic-specific antigen (PSA) measurement, and transrectal prostate ultrasonography and biopsies in selected cases as appropriate.

Diagnostic modalities: DRE, PSA and transrectal ultrasound-directed prostatic biopsy

Digital rectal examination and serum PSA are the most useful first-line tests for assessing an individual (Catalona *et al.* 1994; Stone *et al.* 1994). The positive predictive value of DRE if cancer is present ranges between 21% and 53% as shown in several studies (Cooner *et al.* 1990; Catalona *et al.* 1994; Ellis *et al.* 1994; Stone *et al.* 1994). It has only a fair reproducibility in experienced hands (Smith & Catalona 1995). Classification of localised untreated prostate cancer (T1 and T2), as seen in Table 5.1, should be the aim of early diagnosis if optimal outcome is to be achieved. It is accepted that a dramatic increase in prostate cancer detection between 1986 and 1991 was due to PSA testing (Demers *et al.* 1994; Potosky *et al.* 1995). Although an abnormal DRE or an elevated PSA may suggest the presence of prostate cancer, this disease can be confirmed only by pathological examination of prostate tissue. Decisions with regard to obtaining biopsies should be individualised, and benefits and consequences should be discussed with the patient before PSA testing and prostatic biopsies.

Table 5.1 Prostate cancer staging using the TNM system (1992 revision)

T1a	< 5% PURP chippings (+) for prostate cancer
T1b	> 5% PURP chippings (+) for prostate cancer
T1c	Impalpable – Prostate cancer found by biopsy
T2a	Palpable nodule < half the prostate lobe involved
T2b	Palpable nodule > half the prostate lobe involved
T2c	Bilateral nodes or one nodule involving both lobes

PURP, periurethral prostatectomy.

The relatively long natural history of most prostate cancers renders early detection non-beneficial in men with limited life expectancy. The main acknowledged factors indicating high-risk patients are men with first-degree relatives who have the disease (Wynder *et al.* 1971; Spitz *et al.* 1991). In addition, ethnic origin is to be positively taken into account because it has been demonstrated that African–American men are at a substantially greater risk of developing the disease, and at an earlier age, compared with other ethnic groups (Ernster et al 1978; Boring *et al.* 1992).

The information derived from biopsies can be extremely valuable in predicting the possible stage and outcome of the disease. It has been demonstrated that the nerve bundle pathways around the prostate gland have two main ports of entry, namely the *superior pedicle nerves*, which encompass up to 80% of the nerves supplying the prostate, and *inferior pedicle nerves*, which encompass up to 20% (McNeal 1992). Perineural invasion in histological evaluation of the specimens obtained has been correlated to capsular penetration in radical prostatectomy specimens (Bastacky *et al.* 1993). It was thought by Villers *et al.* (1989) that nerves penetrating the capsule would provide the path of least resistance. Capsular penetration has been proposed by Stamey *et al.* (1988, 1989) to play a major role in deciding the outcome of treatment of the disease. Focal or limited penetration is usually linked to excellent prognosis. However, complete capsular penetration, where there is more than 1 cm from the capsule involved with tumour, carries a poor prognosis. The extent of capsular penetration and the possible risk of involvement of the regional lymph nodes and seminal vesicles are shown in Figure 5.2. Partin *et al.* (1997) indicated that a combination of PSA value, clinical stage and the histological Gleason score is valuable in predicting the pathological stage of localised prostate cancer. This was based on multi-institutional data collection, which is now accepted as the basis of counselling between the treating urologist and his patient with regard to the possible outcome of radical prostatectomy. The relationship between these factors and capsular penetration is shown in Figure 5.3. Roach (1993) and Roach *et al.* (1994) provided a formula assessing the possibility of capsular penetration, seminal vesicle invasion

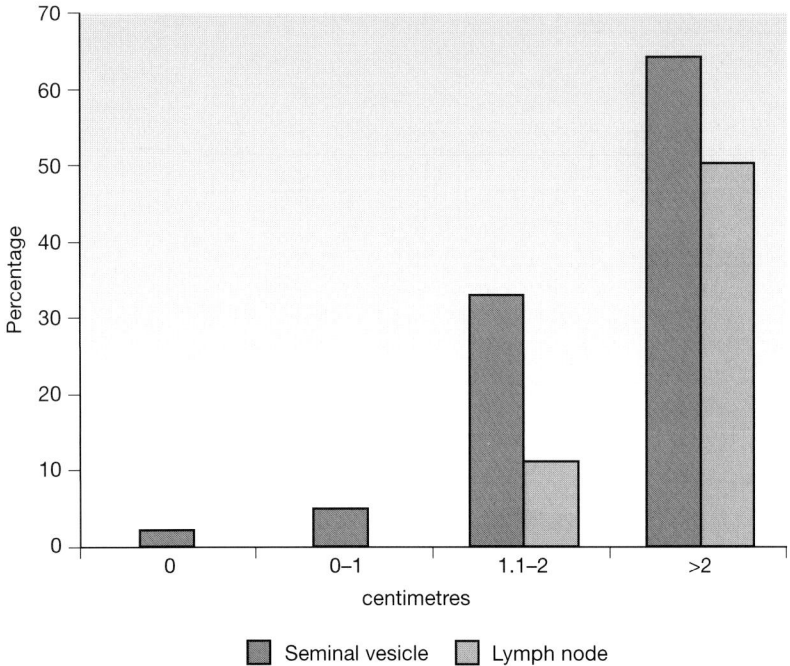

Figure 5.2 Extent of capsular penetration and risk of seminal vesicle or lymph node involvement.

and lymph node involvement, taking into account the PSA reading and Gleason scoring of the biopsies. It was in agreement with Partin's tables as well. The term 'extraprostatic extension' was accepted in 1996 to replace other terms, including 'capsular invasion' 'capsular penetration' and 'capsular perforation' (Sakr *et al.* 1996). A detailed description of the anatomy of the capsule was published in detail in 1998 by Bostwick and Foster.

In patients undergoing radical prostatectomy, the full evaluation of the specimen identifies three different groups of patients. Group 1 has a lower-risk outcome where the total volume of the tumour is less than 3–4 cm³. Group 2 has an intermediate risk, where the volume of the tumour is 3.5–12.0 cm³. Group 3 represents the high-risk group, where the tumour volume is more than 12 cm³. Tumours in the peripheral zone are not as preferable as those in the transition zone. These findings could be of an immense value in counselling newly diagnosed patients with regard to the overall outcome of their disease.

Quality of life – sequelae of radical prostatectomy

Surgical treatment of localised prostatic carcinoma has raised much debate concerning urinary incontinence, sexual dysfunction and global satisfaction. These are the main points of debate on which the patient's decision is taken. In a recent

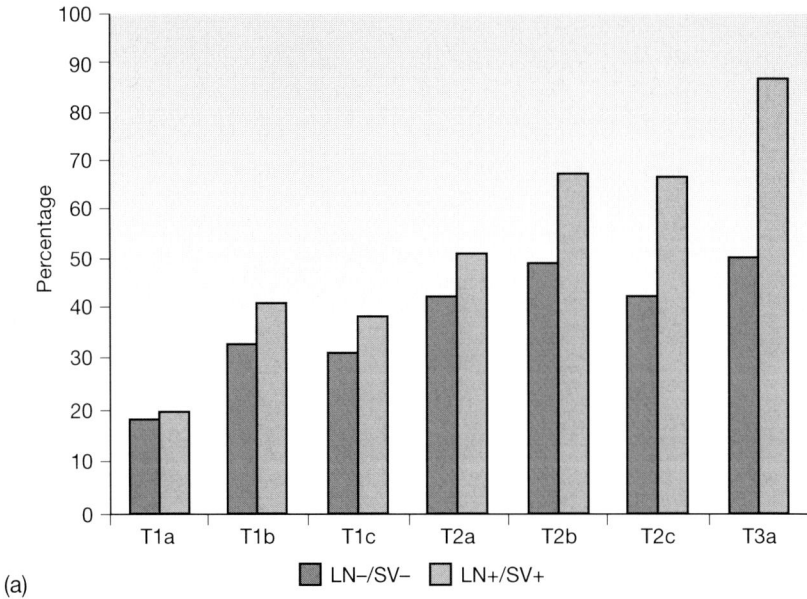

(a)

LN–/SV–   LN+/SV+

Figure 5.3 Relationship between different factors and capsular penetration.
(a) Clinical stage and capsular penetration; (b) PSA and capsular penetration;
(c) Gleason score and capsular penetration.

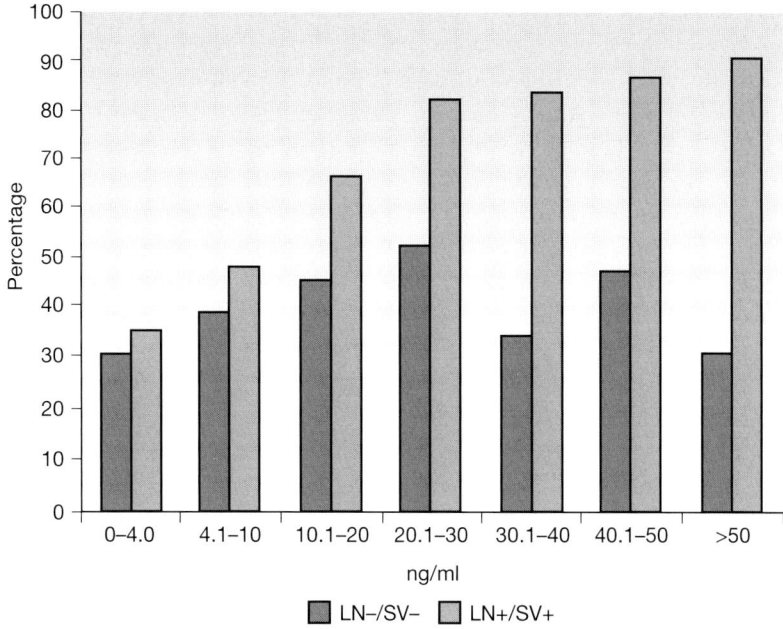

(b)

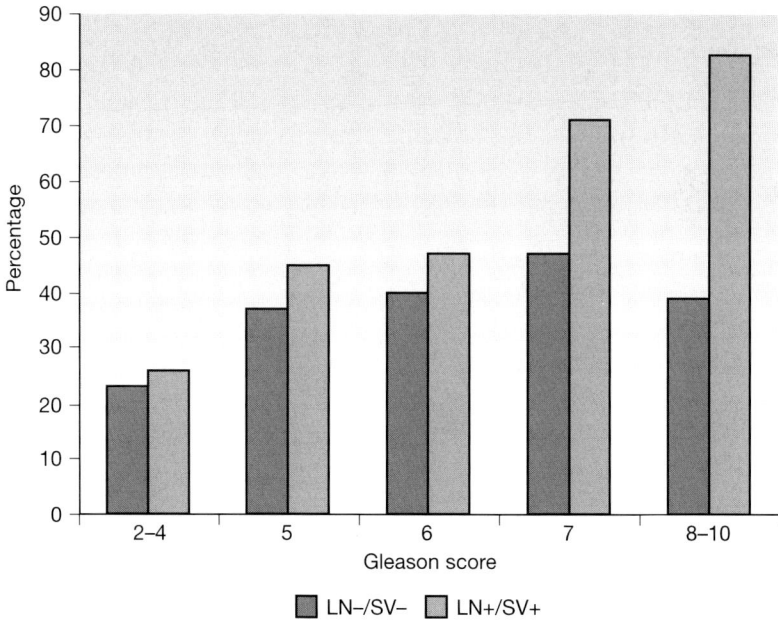

(c)

Figure 5.3 contd

report by Potosky *et al.* (2000) urinary function, sexual domain and overall satisfaction were discussed. The report based its findings on an average practice, rather than the highly specialised unit, which would provide benchmark outcomes. Undoubtedly, results of urinary function assessment improve in a particular unit. The sexual domain items were debated and it was noted that younger patients experienced a greater improvement in sexual function during the second year. The level of pre-treatment sexual dysfunction has not really been well rehearsed, which would have an impact on the post-treatment results. There are aids available to help patients to achieve satisfactory sexual function, namely pharmacological injectable/intracavitary measures, vacuum constriction devices and penile implants. Understanding the anatomical pathway of the neurovascular bundle has led recently to attempted usage of peroperative nerve stimulation in an attempt to improve the nerve-sparing modification of radical prostatectomy. However, there was an interesting debate about the value of such a device, indicating that the results are not yet conclusive. Although Klotz *et al.* (2000) reported the results of a randomised phase III study of intraoperative cavernous nerve stimulation with penile tumescence monitoring, deeming it useful, Kim *et al.* (2000) reported that a positive response poorly predicted the recovery of potency after radical prostatectomy. The plethora of quality-of-life outcome studies in patients with prostate cancer receiving various treatment modalities are a long way off being conclusive. It is interesting that some patients, up to 91%, longing for a cure of the disease indicate that maintenance of sexual activity is of less importance (Rosetti & Terrone 1996).

Conclusion

Although there is a lack of prospective randomised studies comparing the efficacy of radical prostatectomy, neoadjuvant external beam radiotherapy and brachytherapy, surgeons are faced with patients who need immediate action taken according to their diagnosis. It is fair to say that urological surgeons have valuable guidelines that would help greatly in selecting patients for radical prostatectomy, and could counsel and offer, to the best of their ability, a prudent estimate of the long-term outcome.

References

Bastacky SI, Walsh PC, Epstein JI *et al.* (1993). Relationship between perineural tumour invasion on needle biopsy and radical prostatectomy capsular penetration in clinical stage B adenocarcinoma of the prostate. *American Journal of Surgical Pathology* **17**, 336–341

Boring CC, Squires TS, Heath CW Jr (1992). Cancer statistics for African Americans. *CA: Cancer Journal for Clinicians* **42**, 7–17

Bostwick CC & Foster CS (1998). Examination of radical prostatectomy specimens, therapeutic and prognostic significance. In: Foster CS & Bostwick CC (eds) *Pathology of the Prostate.* Philadelphia: WB Saunders Co., pp 172–189

Bostwick DG (1999). Prostatic intraepithelial neoplasia. In: Kaisary AV, Murphy PG, Denis L, Griffiths K (eds*) Textbook of Prostate Cancer, Pathology, Diagnosis and Treatment,* 1st edn. London: Martin Dunitz Ltd, pp 35–50

Catalona WJ, Ritchie JP, Ahmann FR *et al.* (1994). Comparison of digital rectal examination and serum prostate specific antigen in the early detection of prostate cancer, Results of a multicenter clinical trial of 6630 men. *Journal of Urology* **151**, 1283–1290

Cooner WH, Mosley BR, Rutherford CL Jr *et al.* (1990). Prostate cancer detection in a clinical urological practice by ultrasonography, digital ractal examination and prostate specific antigen. *Journal of Urology* **143**, 1146–1154

Demers RY, Swanson GM, Weiss LK *et al.* (1994). Increasing incidence of cancer of the prostate.The experience of black and white men in the Detroit metropolitan area. *Archives of Internal Medicine* **154**, 1211–1216

Ellis WJ, Chetner MP, Preston SD, Brawer MK (1994). Diagnosis of prostatic carcinoma, The yield of serum prostate specific antigen, digital rectal examination and transrectal ultrasonography. *Journal of Urology* **152**, 1520–1525

Ernster VL, Selvin S, Sacks ST *et al.* (1978). Prostatic cancer, Mortality and incidence rates by race and social class. *American Journal of Epidemiology* **107**, 311–320

Kim HL, Stoffel DS, Mhoon D *et al.* (2000). A positive CaverMap response poorly predicts recovery of potency after radical prostatectomy. *Urology* **56**, 561–564

Klotz L, Heaton J, Jewett M *et al.* (2000). A randomised phase 3 study of intraoperative cavernous nerve stimulation with penile tumescence monitoring to improve nerve sparing during radical prostatectomy. *Journal of Urology* **164**, 1573–1578

McNeal JE (1992). Cancer volume and site of origin of adenocarcinoma in the prostate, relationship to local and distant spread. *Human Pathology* **23**, 258–266

Office for National Statistics (2000). *Expectation of Life at Selected Ages by Gender, 1911 to 2021 (Selected Years).* Social Trends Dataset

Partin AW, Kattan MW, Subong EN *et al.* (1997). Combination of Prostate Specific Antigen, Clinical Stage and Gleason Score to predict pathological stage of localised prostate cancer. *Journal of the American Medical Association* **277**, 1445–1451

Potosky AL, Miller BA, Albertsen PC *et al.* (1995). The role of increasing detection in the rising incidence of prostate cancer. *Journal of the American Medical Association* **273**, 548–552

Potosky AL, Legler J, Albertsen PC *et al.* (2000). Health Outcomes After Prostatectomy or Radiotherapy for Prostate Cancer, Results from the Prostate Cancer Outcome Study. *Journal of the National Cancer Institute* **92**, 1582–1592

Roach M (1993). The use of prostate specific antigen, clinical stage and Gleason score to predict pathological stage in men with localised prostate cancer. *Journal of Urology* **150**, 1923–1924

Roach M, Marquez C, You HS *et al.* (1994). Predicting the risk of lymph node involvement using the pre-treatment prostate specific antigen and Gleason score in men with clinically localised prostate cancer. *International Journal of Radiation Oncology* **28**, 33–37

Rossetti SR & Terrone C (1996). Quality of life in prostate cancer patients. *European Urology* **30**, 44–48

Sakr W, Wheeler T, Blute M *et al.* (1996). Staging and reporting of prostate cancer. Sampling of the radical prostatectomy specimens. *Cancer* **78**, 366–368

Smith DS & Catalona WJ (1995). Interexaminer variability of digital rectal examination in detecting prostate cancer. *Urology* **45**, 70–74

Spitz MR, Currier RD, Fueger JJ *et al.* (1991). Familial patterns of prostate cancer, A case-control analysis. *Journal of Urology* **146**, 1305–1307

Stamey TA, McNeal JE, Freiha FS *et al.* (1988). Morphometric and clinical studies on 68 consecutive radical prostatectomies. *Journal of Urology* **139**, 1235–1241

Stamey TA, Kabalin JN, McNeal JE *et al.* (1989). Prostate specific antigen in the diagnosis and treatment of adenocarcinoma of the prostate. II. Radical prostatectomy patients. *Journal of Urology* **141**, 1076–1083

Stone NN, DeAntoni EP, Crawford ED (1994). Screening for prostate cancer by digital rectal examination and prostate-specific antigen, Results of prostate cancer awareness week, 1989–1992. *Urology* **44**, 18–25

Villers A, McNeal JE, Redwine EA *et al.* (1989). The role of perineural space invasion in the local spread of prostatic adenocarcinoma. *Journal of Urology* **142**, 763–768

Wynder EL, Mabuchi K, Whitmore WF Jr (1971). Epidemiology of cancer of the prostate. *Cancer* **28**, 344–360

Clinical utility of external beam radiotherapy alone or in combination with hormone treatment for localised disease

David P Dearnaley

Introduction

Controversy will continue to surround the optimal individual management of localised prostate cancer until we have more accurate tools to predict both the local behaviour and the metastatic potential of the disease. At present it seems reasonable to offer curative treatment to men judged to have a life expectancy of 10 years or more, although this may be modified to 5 years for men who have poorly differentiated cancers (Dearnaley & Melia 1997; Lu Yao & Yao 1997). The relative merits of radical radiotherapy or surgery depend on both local tumour control probability and treatment-induced morbidity. No adequate studies have compared these treatment alternatives and both should be considered as standard management options for patients with disease confined to the prostate (Consensus Conference 1987; COIN Guidelines 1999).

In North America radical prostatectomy is now the most commonly used radical treatment option for localised disease, although radiotherapy is given to approximately 30% of patients. In the UK radiotherapy is used most frequently although precise figures are not available. The comparisons that have been made between the two options suggest that there is little difference in outcome (D'Amico *et al.* 1997). It can be argued that success or failure of treatment is more dependent on tumour biology than the treatment method and that of treatment-related morbidity as much on the skill of the individual specialist as on the treatment modality employed. There has been considerable development of radiotherapy techniques and strategies over the last 10 years. Conformal radiotherapy has now become the standard of care as a result of prospective phase III randomised trials. Initial (neoadjuvant) hormone therapy is widely employed and has been shown to improve both local and biochemical control of disease. Studies of adjuvant hormonal treatment and radiotherapy have additionally shown that there is a survival advantage for longer-term androgen suppression for men with more advanced, poorly differentiated cancers. Sophisticated radiotherapy techniques now allow high doses of radiation to be given and preliminary results strongly suggest improved control rates with very acceptable levels of long-term morbidity. Prostate-specific antigen (PSA) testing can be expected to have a very major impact on the stage of disease at presentation (Hankey *et al.* 1999). Patients with small PSA-detected cancers (T1c) can be expected to have a much more favourable outcome than men with more advanced, clinically diagnosed T2–T3 cancers, which remains the predominant presentation in the UK. If more men with early localised disease are to receive treatment, it is of course mandatory that this be given with the minimum possible side effects.

Selection of patients for radical radiotherapy

Radical radiotherapy should be reserved for those patients presenting without evidence of distant metastasis. The prognosis of patients with incidental (T1a), focal, well-differentiated disease is so good (Lowe & Linstrom 1988) that immediate treatment is difficult to justify. Patients with T1b, T1c and T2–T3 disease are suitable for radical treatment depending on their age and general state of health. The decision to offer treatment is based on a judgement of the balance between the life expectancy of an individual patient and a chance of their disease progressing during this period of time. The seminal article by Chodak *et al.* (1994) has shown that tumour grade is of overriding importance in determining outcome for men with T1 and T2 cancers. For well, moderately and poorly differentiated cancers the rates of developing metastasis at 10 years were 19%, 41% and 74% respectively, and 13% of men with grade 1/2 tumours died from prostate cancer at 10 years compared to 66% of men with grade 3 cancers. The probability of curative treatment is high for small-volume, relatively well-differentiated cancers. As tumour bulk increases so does the chance of seminal vesicle or lymph node involvement, and patients with lymph node involvement have a 75% chance of developing metastatic disease within 5 years (Perez *et al.* 1989).

Computed tomography (CT) or magnetic resonance imaging (MRI) are now the imaging methods of choice for determining the presence or absence of lymph node involvement, although false-negative results are common. In selected cases mini-laparotomy or laparoscopic lymph node devaluation can be justified. If lymph node involvement is shown then radical local treatment (with surgery or radiotherapy) is inappropriate when used alone, although there is some evidence that combination with long-term androgen suppression may give improved results (see below). The PSA level at presentation also gives a valuable guide to probable treatment outcome (Shipley *et al.* 1999; Kattan *et al.* 2000). Currently tumour stage, histological grade (usually the Gleason score) and presenting PSA levels are very commonly used to stratify patients to receive neoadjuvant or adjuvant hormonal therapy in addition to modifying radiation dosage.

Results of radical external beam radiotherapy alone

After external beam radiotherapy, long-term clinically assessed control of local tumours is good for patients with stage T1 cancers (83% at 15 years), but becomes less secure with increasing T stage, falling to 65–68% for T2 and 44–75% for T3 cancers (Table 6.1). Larger cancers have higher failure rates, rising from 25% for tumours palpably $\leq$ 25 cm^2 to more than 50% for tumours with a product of their diameter > 25 cm^2 (Pilepich *et al.* 1987). Previously, most local recurrences have been detected by digital rectal examination (DRE) and the true rate determined by post-irradiation biopsy is probably higher. There is general agreement that a positive biopsy 24 months after radiotherapy indicates persisting disease (Crook *et al.* 1993). The reported rates of positive biopsy vary considerably and the true incidence of positive biopsy results in patients with normal DRE is uncertain (Zietman *et al.* 1993). Reported incidence of positive biopsy vary from 18 to 45% after treatment and increases with disease bulk from 15% for men with B1 disease (< 1.5-cm nodule) to 68–79% for men with bulky stage B or C cancers (Freiha & Bagshaw 1984; Scardino & Bretas 1987).

Table 6.1 External beam radiotherapy for cancer of the prostate: long-term results from patterns of care surveys, radiotherapy and oncology group studies and large single institute series

No.	Local recurrence rate (%)			Survival rate with no evidence of disease (%)			Overall survival rate (%)		
	5 yrs	10 yrs	15 yrs	5 yrs	10 yrs	15 yrs	5 yrs	10 yrs	15 yrs
T1NX 583	3–6	4–8	17	84–85	52–68	39	83–95	52–76	41–46
T2NX 1,117	12–14	17–29	32–35	66–90	27–85	15–42	74–78	43–70	22–36
T3NX 2,292	12–26	19–31	25–56	32–60	14–46	17–40	56–72	32–42	23–27

Sources: Pilepich *et al.* (1987); Zagars *et al.* (1987); Perez *et al.* (1988); Goffinet and Baghaw (1990).

It has become clear that PSA estimation both before and after irradiation can give very useful prognostic information to guide selection of patients for treatment, as well as being a very sensitive indicator of disease recurrence. Hanks *et al.* (1996a) studied 110 patients with T1–T3 prostate cancer with a mean follow-up of 12.6 years and found long-term biochemical control in 72% of T1 cancers, 54% of T2A cancers, falling to 22% and 28% for bulky T2 and T3 cancers, respectively. Favourable outcome was also seen in cancers of low Gleason score which had a 75% rate of biochemical control compared with only 18% for Gleason 7 and 0% of Gleason 8 or 9 carcinomas. We have also learnt that pre-treatment PSA levels are of critical importance (Shipley *et al.* 1992; Hanks *et al.* 1996b, 1998; Zelefsky *et al.* 1998; Kattan *et al.* 2000), e.g. Hanks *et al.* found that for 120 patients with PSA > 20 ng/ml at presentation only 28% remained biochemically free of progressive disease at 4 years, although 81% still had no evidence of distant metastasis, which suggests that locoregional recurrence may be a major component of disease failure.

A recent multi-institutional pooled analysis (Shipley *et al.* 1999) has reported on a total of 1,765 men with stage T1b, T1c and T2 tumours. They found that presenting

PSA level was a powerful predictor of outcome and the estimated rates of remaining free of biochemical (PSA) recurrence according to pre-treatment PSA values were 81%, 68%, 51% and 31% for men presenting with pre-treatment PSA values of < 10 ng/ml, 10–20 ng/ml, 20–30 ng/ml and > 30 ng/ml respectively. These results are currently a benchmark against which other treatment approaches should be measured. Another important conclusion from this study was that biochemical or clinical recurrence was unlikely more than 5 years after treatment (95% of patients remained free from failure if PSA levels were controlled at 5 years) and this result has been substantiated by other authors (Hanlon & Hanks 2000; Vicini *et al.* 2000).

Complications after conventional external beam radiotherapy

Radiation-induced complications are dose limiting, and conventional radiotherapy doses and fractionation schedules have been derived from years of clinical experience to give acceptable morbidity. Acute side effects from radiotherapy to the pelvis include acute proctitis causing rectal discomfort and diarrhoea, acute cystitis producing dysuria and urinary frequency, and occasional skin reactions (Amdur *et al.* 1990; Mithal & Hoskin 1990; Duncan *et al.* 1993). Reported incidence ranges between 70 and 90% for mild symptoms, 20 and 45% for moderate, and 1 and 4% for severe or prolonged reactions. Such side effects depend on the volume of tissue irradiated (e.g. pelvis and prostate or prostate only) (Sagerman *et al.* 1989) and also relate to the treatment technique. Acute side effects are expected to settle within 4–6 weeks of completing radiotherapy.

Late complications may develop months to years after treatment and are potentially of more concern. Late gastrointestinal side effects include persistent rectal discharge, tenesmus and rectal urgency, rectal bleeding, ulcer or stricture. Important late genitourinary complications include chronic cystitis, bladder ulcer, urinary incontinence, urethral stricture and impotence.

Results from over 1,000 patients treated in a single institute series suggest an overall moderate complication rate of 16–19%, with severe complications requiring surgical correction in 1–3% of cases (Aristizabal *et al.* 1984; Forman *et al.* 1985; Zagars *et al.* 1987). Poor treatment technique and doses above 70 Gy were also associated with increased complications (Leibel *et al.* 1984). With a 10-year follow-up, 2% of patients had needed surgical correction of complications, a further 2% had developed a major complication not requiring surgery, and two patients had died from treatment-related side effects. The actuarial 5- and 10-year complication-free survival rates were 93% and 86% respectively (Hanks *et al.* 1987). An increase in the overall complication rate from 6 to 11% was noted for patients treated with doses below and above 65 Gy respectively (Hanks *et al.* 1988a). The remaining complication is impotence, which has been estimated to occur in between 30 and 40% of treated men, usually during the 6 months after treatment (De Wit *et al.* 1983). In a recent Radiotherapy and Oncology Group (RTOG) randomised study (Pilepich *et al.* 1995),

76% of men who were sexually potent before treatment reported return of sexual function. In a report of conformal therapy (Roach *et al*. 1996), 62% of men reported return of sexual function. However, patients have consistently reported a higher level of morbidity than may be appreciated from scales of physician-based reporting (Potosky *et al*. 2000). This very comprehensive (but not randomised) study showed that, compared with baseline, radiotherapy had a minimal effect on urinary function in contradistinction to total prostatectomy, although radiotherapy produced more bowel disturbance. After surgery 12% of men were bothered (reporting a big or moderate problem) by urinary leaking or dripping compared with 2% of men after radiotherapy. Conversely, 6% of men reported bother after radiotherapy from increased bowel movements, pain or urgency compared with 4% of men after surgery. For men between the ages of 55 and 59 years, 75% were bothered by sexual dysfunction after surgery compared with 40% after radiotherapy; for those aged between 60 and 74 figures were 53% and 47% respectively 2 years after treatment. Global measures of quality of life appear to be affected little by treatment (Widmark *et al*. 1994; Litwin *et al*. 1995; Roach *et al*. 1996; Beard *et al*. 1997; Potosky *et al*. 2000).

Approaches to improve the results of radiotherapy

Although radical radiotherapy is successful in obtaining clinically judged local control of disease in the majority of patients with T1–T3 disease, the development of metastatic disease is a major problem particularly for more bulky disease presentations and for those cancers with high presenting PSA levels or poorly differentiated pathology.

There is now considerable circumstantial evidence that failure to gain local control of disease is associated with an increased rate of development of distant metastasis. A review of our own patients at Royal Marsden Hospital showed 57% metastasis-free survival at 5 years in patients with clinically locally controlled disease compared with 26% of patients with local recurrence ($p < 0.01$), and local control remained highly significant ($p < 0.001$) when included as a time-dependent variable in a multivariate analysis of survival and metastases-free survival. These findings are in accord with other series that have documented distant metastases developing in 19–41% of patients with stages A–C disease who have had their local disease controlled, compared with 57–83% for similar patients who have developed local failure (Leibel *et al*. 1994). Local failure has been reported to be the most important determinant on multivariate analysis in predicting the development of metastatic disease (Fuks *et al*. 1991); Yorke *et al*. (1993) estimated, using Monte Carlo simulation techniques, that 50% of metastases in patients with local recurrence were the result of local treatment failure.

Different but complementary approaches are being developed to improve results using radiotherapy (Table 6.2). These are either methods (1) to improve the local control of disease increasing radiation dose in a variety of ways or employing the initial use of neoadjuvant hormone therapy or (2) that use systemic adjuvant androgen

Table 6.2 Methods to improve results of radical radiotherapy for prostate cancer

	Improve local control	*Reduce risk of development of metastases*
Increase dose	Conformal radiotherapy Intensity-modulated radiotherapy Brachytherapy Particle beam therapy	Systemic treatment: androgen blockade
		Reduce local treatment failure
Neoadjuvant hormonal therapy		

blockade (an analogy can be made with the use of tamoxifen in breast cancer) to reduce the risk of development of metastasis.

Conformal radiotherapy

As described previously, the complication rate from standard prostate radiotherapy increases with increasing dose so that doses above 65–70 Gy are associated with unacceptable complications. The principal dose-limiting late complication is proctitis caused by radiation of the rectum. Nevertheless, retrospective data have shown improvement in local control using higher doses of radiation, e.g. the Patterns of Care Studies Group (Hanks *et al*. 1988b) reported results from 1,348 men with stage B and C cancers. The actuarial 5-year local recurrence rate for stage C disease was 37% for doses < 60 Gy, 36% for 64–66 Gy, 28% for 65–69 Gy and 19% for doses > 70 Gy. Dose escalation therefore seems justified.

Conformal radiotherapy is a new technology developed over the last 10 years or more to enable radiation fields to be shaped accurately to follow the outline of the target tissues. The process involves, first, the three-dimensional visualisation of target structures, in this case prostate with or without seminal vesicles. This is achieved using closely collimated CT slices, which are then reconstructed in three dimensions so that shaped rather than the conventional rectangular radiation beams can encompass the target. There have been considerable developments in radiotherapy outlining and planning software so that these procedures can now be undertaken rapidly and routinely. The radiation beams are most conveniently shape with a multileaf collimator which is routinely installed on most new linear accelerators. Verification of accuracy is a very important part of the process and this can be ensured by taking electronic portal images of the radiotherapy treatment fields, which can be directly compared with simulator films or ideally digitally reconstructed radiographs from the original CT images. Using these methods the amount of excess normal tissue treated is reduced by approximately 50%. Conformal and conventional radiotherapy for prostate cancer have been formally compared in a prospective phase III trial using a standard radiation dose of 64 Gy (Dearnaley *et al*. 1999). Men were randomly allocated to conformal or conventional radiotherapy treatments. Significantly fewer developed radiation-induced proctitis and bleeding in the conformal group than in the conventional group (37% vs 56% ≥ RTOG grade 1, $p = 0.004$; 5% vs 15% ≥ RTOG grade 2, $p = 0.01$). After a median follow-up of 3.6 years, there was no difference between the groups in local tumour control. This study has laid a firm scientific foundation for the introduction of conformal radiotherapy in routine practice and also for escalating dose using conformal radiotherapy techniques.

Dose-escalation studies using three-dimensional conformal radiotherapy (3DCRT) have been reported by several North American groups (Sandler *et al.* 1992; Hanks *et al.* 1998; Zelefsky *et al.* 1998). Zelefesky *et al.* (1998) reported that complete response (defined as PSA ≤ 1.0 ng/ml) occurred in 90% in patients receiving 75.6 Gy or 81 Gy, compared with 76% and 56% for those treated to 70.2 Gy and 64.8 Gy respectively ($p < 0.001$). Five-year actuarial PSA relapse-free survival was significantly improved in patients with intermediate or unfavourable prognosis receiving ≥ 75.6 Gy ($p < 0.05$). The positive biopsy rate at 2.5 years or longer after 3DCRT was 7% in patients receiving 81 Gy, 48% after 75.6 Gy, 45% after 70.2 Gy and 57% after 64.8 Gy ($p < 0.05$), although the number of patients was small. In addition, Hanks *et al.* (1998) have reported that, in patients with initial PSA ≥ 10 ng/ml, 2-year PSA control rates were 85% for patients who received more than 71 Gy compared with 72% for those who received lower doses ($p = 0.007$). Similarly a recent multi-institutional review (Fiveash *et al.* 2000) demonstrated improved biochemical control 5 years after treatment completion for high-grade T1 and T2 cancers treated to a dose of > 70 Gy. The first report of an overall improvement in survival has come from the North American RTOG (Valicenti *et al.* 2000). Pooled data from 1,465 men treated in RTOG studies showed that, for men with high-grade cancers, a higher radiation dose (≥ 66 Gy versus ≤ 66 Gy) was associated with a 29% lower risk of death from prostate cancer and a 27% reduction in overall mortality rate ($p < 0.05$). A substantial body of data from randomised control trials of dose escalation will become available within the next few years. The first trial to report was performed by the MD Anderson Cancer Centre. They randomised a total of 305 men to receive either 70 Gy delivered using conventional radiotherapy techniques or 78 Gy using conformal radiotherapy methods. The failure-free survival rates at 5 years were 69% and 79% respectively ($p = 0.06$) with multivariate analysis showing significant benefit for men with a presenting PSA level of > 10 ng/ml (Pollack *et al.* 2000).

In the UK, a large randomised trial will complete recruitment in 2001. After a pilot study undertaken at the Institute of Cancer Research and the Royal Marsden Hospital, a total of over 900 men will be randomised to receive either 64 Gy or 74 Gy using conformal radiotherapy methods after initial androgen suppression for 3–6 months (Seddon *et al.* 2000). A complementary study undertaken by the National Cancer Institute in Amsterdam will randomise approximately 600 men to receive either 70 Gy or 78 Gy, again using conformal radiotherapy techniques in both arms of the study. Meta-analysis of these and additional trials will, in due course, adequately define the role of dose escalation in different subgroups of patients, assessing overall and disease-specific survival benefits – as well as impact on PSA control and treatment-related side effects. The importance of maintaining therapy-related morbidity to a minimum is essential. Already the Memorial Sloane Kettering group has shown that, with very meticulous technique and scrupulous shielding of the rectum, it is possible to treat patients to between 75 and 81 Gy with a low rate of long-term rectal complications (Zelefsky *et al.* 2000), and using very sophisticated intensity-modulated radiotherapy techniques this group have reported a 2-year actuarial risk of grade 2 bleeding and proctitis of only 2%.

It will be a challenge for the radiotherapy community to implement such methods routinely.

Combined modality treatment using androgen suppression and radiotherapy

Laboratory and both preliminary and phase III randomised clinical trials have now demonstrated clear advantages from using combinations of hormonal therapy with radiotherapy in the management of localised prostate cancer. Hormonal treatment can be given before radiation for a period of 2–6 months or more (neoadjuvant therapy), or alternatively it may be used in an adjuvant fashion continuing after radiotherapy for periods of 2 years or more. Neoadjuvant hormonal therapy is complementary to attempts to improve results of radiotherapy using conformal radiotherapy with or without dose escalation (Figure 6.1). However, we have not yet learnt what is the optimal combination of these different approaches. The precise definition of groups of patients that may benefit from adjuvant treatment is also currently unclear, although both of these issues will be resolved as data from current phase III studies become available.

Combined modality treatment has been studied in animal models. Using a transplantable tumour in athymic nude mice (Zietman *et al.* 1997), orchiectomy performed 12 days before radiation (neoadjuvant therapy) reduced the TCD_{50} (dose that controls 50% of tumours) from 86 Gy for radiotherapy alone to 43 Gy for neoadjuvant orchiectomy and radiotherapy. Interestingly, however, orchiectomy performed 1–12 days after irradiation (adjuvant therapy) had a much smaller effect (TCD_{50} of 69 Gy and 75 Gy respectively). In a rat prostate tumour model androgen ablation 3 days before radiotherapy increased the apoptotic index by five- to tenfold compared with controls. However, when irradiation was commenced at the same time as androgen ablation, no supra-additive effect was seen (Joon *et al.* 1997). These studies suggest that the timing and sequencing of combined hormonal treatments and radiotherapy may be critical to obtain optimal results.

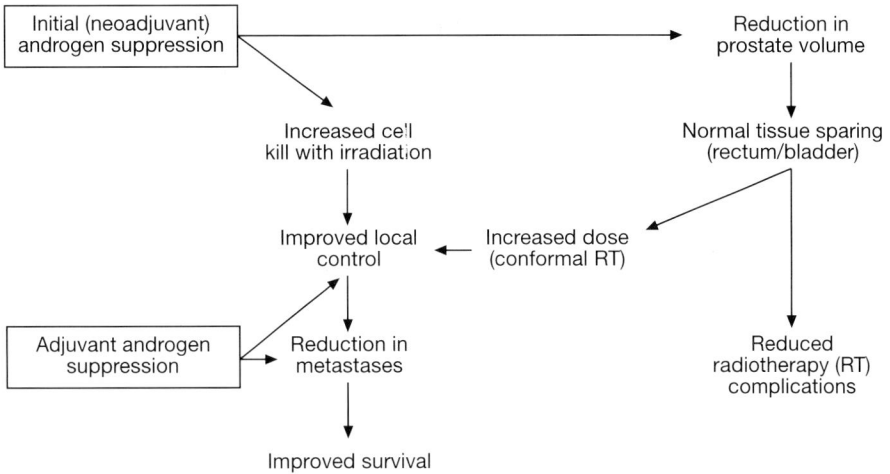

Figure 6.1 Combined modality treatment using androgen suppression and radiotherapy.

Clinical studies of neoadjuvant androgen suppression and radiotherapy

Combined modality treatment using initial hormones followed by radiotherapy can potentially have advantages in two ways (see Figure 6.1). First, the prostate and radiotherapy target volume may be decreased leading to a benefit in therapeutic ratio and, second, as in the experimental models there may be an additive or supra-additive effect on prostate cancer cell death. Different groups of researchers have shown very similar results for reduction of prostate radiotherapy target volumes. At the Royal Marsden Hospital, 22 patients were treated with 3–6 months of androgen suppression using a luteinising hormone-releasing hormone analogue (LHRHa) before radiotherapy. Monthly transrectal ultrasonic measurements were made and the prostate volume reduced by approximately 50% (Shearer *et al.* 1992), the median pre-treatment volume of 66 ml (range 40–130 ml) reducing to 30 ml (range 30–47 ml). Notably, most patients had significant improvements in symptoms of ordinary outflow obstruction before radiotherapy. Radiotherapy planning CT scans were taken before and after hormonal therapy and a 41% reduction in radiotherapy target volume was shown, with 22% and 43% reductions in the rectal and bladder volumes, respectively, treated to high dose (Dearnaley 2000). Similarly, Forman *et al.* (1995) reported an average 37% reduction in prostate volume after 3 months of hormonal therapy, with 23% reduction in the volume of rectum and 21% reduction of the volume of bladder receiving 64 Gy; Zelefsky *et al.* (1994) showed a mean 25% reduction in target volume with 25% and 50% reductions in volumes of rectum and bladder treated.

Phase III trials of initial hormonal treatment and radiotherapy

Three phase III trials have now reported the results of comparisons of radiotherapy with or without neoadjuvant androgen deprivation. The first and largest undertaken by the RTOG randomised 471 patients with large primary tumours (T2–T4) and no evidence of distant metastases to receive maximal androgen blockade using goserelin and flutamide 2 months before and during radiation treatment (group I) or radiotherapy alone (group II) (Pilepich *et al.* 1995). The most recently reported results show highly significant benefits in 5-year rates of local disease control (group I 75%, group II 64%, $p = 0.002$), freedom from distance metastases (group I 71%, group II 61%, $p = 0.03$), and no evidence of disease including PSA failure (group I 39%, group II 20%, $p < 0.0001$). After 8 years of follow-up, there is a suggestion that the survival in group I (51%) may be improved compared with group II (42%), although this result does not reach statistical significance ($p = 0.2$) (Pilepich *et al.* 1998). In a similar but smaller Canadian Urological Oncology Group study, 208 patients with stage B2–C prostate cancer were randomly allocated to a 12-week initial course of cyproterone acetate followed by radiotherapy (group I) or radiotherapy alone (group II). On average the PSA nadir was lower in the combined modality group and more patients (group I) remained free of clinical (71% vs 49%, $p = 0.02$) or biochemical (47% vs 22%, $p = 0.001$) recurrence; in addition, after 18 months there was a significant improvement in the number of patients who had negative post-treatment prostate biopsies (Porter *et al.* 1998). In a small three-arm randomised study from Quebec (Laverdiere *et al.* 1997), 120 patients were randomised to receive radiotherapy alone, radiotherapy with an initial 3-month course of maximum androgen blockade or maximum androgen blockade for a total of 11 months. Two-year post-treatment biopsy results showed residual cancer in 65%, 28% and 5% of these three groups, respectively.

Taken together, these three clinical studies provide very strong evidence that initial androgen suppression improves the local control that can be achieved with radiation treatment, and the finding that metastases are reduced indicates that the natural history of the disease is favourably modified. In consequence initial hormone treatment has become the standard of care for appropriate subgroups of men with localised prostate cancer (see below) and is being studied in combination with conformal radiotherapy techniques in the current Medical Research Council (MRC) RT01 Trial (Seddon *et al.* 2000). Although we have demonstrated that testosterone levels recover to the normal range in more than 90% of men who are treated with initial androgen suppression (Dearnaley 2000), impotence may be more common after combined modality treatment (Zelefsky *et al.* 1998). The relative effects of combined modality treatment or high-dose radiotherapy require further study. It is also possible that anti-androgen monotherapy with, for example, bicalutamide may in the future give a more acceptable side-effect profile.

Adjuvant androgen deprivation in combination with radiotherapy

The rational for long-term adjuvant androgen ablation is to employ treatments that demonstrate 'spatial co-operation' in an attempt to treat micrometastatic disease effectively beyond the scope of a local treatment modality. This approach is now well accepted, e.g. in the management of localised breast cancer where adjuvant hormone therapy produces a significant benefit for both recurrence and survival.

In prostate cancer, five randomized controlled trials have reported results. The largest of these was performed by the RTOG (Protocol 85–31) in which 977 men were randomised to receive either radiotherapy to the prostate and pelvis, or radiotherapy and androgen deprivation (Pilepich *et al.* 1997). Hormonal treatment was given using an LHRHa which commenced during the last week of radiotherapy and continued indefinitely. The control group commenced goserelin at the time of relapse. Eligible patients had T3 disease or T1–T2 disease with lymph node involvement. Post-prostectomy patients with adverse features were also eligible. The trial has recently been updated with a median follow-up of 6 years (Lawton *et al.* 2001). Eight-year actuarial results showed significant differences between the groups in local treatment failure (23% vs 37%, $p < 0.0001$), development of distance metastases (27% vs 37%, $p < 0.0001$) as well as biochemical control of disease. Overall survival was not statistically different between the two groups with 49% vs 47% survival at 8 years, but subgroup analysis showed that patients with high-grade (Gleason 8–10) cancers had a statistically significant improvement of both absolute ($p = 0.036$) and cause-specific survival ($p = 0.019$) if adjuvant hormonal therapy had been given. The European Organization for Research and Treatment of Cancer (EORTC) have reported a similar study in which 415 men with either T3–T4 cancers or poorly differentiated T1–T2 tumours were randomised between radiotherapy to the prostate and pelvis alone and combined modality treatment with an LHRHa that was started at the beginning of radiotherapy and continued for a period of 3 years (Bolla *et al.* 1997). Median follow-up at the time of reporting was 45 months. As in the RTOG study, results demonstrated an improvement in local disease control (77% vs 97%, $p < 0.001$), and patients surviving free of disease (48% vs 85%, $p < 0.001$), but also dramatic overall improvement in survival, with 52% of the radiation-alone control group alive at 5 years compared with 79% of the combined modality group ($p = 0.001$). It is possible that the differences between the results of the RTOG and EORTC studies are the result of patient selection, the play of chance or timing of hormonal treatment both before and after radiotherapy.

In a small Swedish Study (Table 6.3), 91 patients were randomised to receive either radiotherapy alone or combined modality treatment with orchiectomy preceding radiotherapy by approximately 6 weeks (Granfors *et al.* 1998). After a median follow-up of 9.3 years, clinical progression was seen in 61% of the radiotherapy-only patients compared with 31% of the combined modality group ($p = 0.005$). Mortality

Table 6.3 Trials of adjuvant hormonal treatment with radiotherapy

Trial identifier	No. of patients	Tumour stage		Randomisation and timing of hormonal treatment
RTOG 85-31	977	A2/B C	D1 D0/1	RT with LHRHa on relapse vs RT + LHRHa starting at end of RT given indefinitely
EORTC 22863	415	T1–T2 T3–T4	G3	RT with LHRHa on relapse vs RT + LHRHa at start of radiotherapy
Sweden	91	T1–T4	N0–N3	RT vs orchidectomy (6 weeks pre-RT) and RT
MRC PRO2	277	T2–T4		Radiotherapy vs orchidectomy and radiotherapy vs orchidectomy
RTOG 92-02	1,554	T2c–T4		Initial androgen suppression + RT vs initial androgen suppression + RT and adjuvant LHRHa for 2 years

LHRHa, luteinising hormone-releasing hormone analogue; RT, radiotherapy.

rates in the two groups were 61% and 38% respectively ($p = 0.02$) with cause-specific mortality rates of 44% and 27% respectively ($p = 0.06$). The MRC have reported results of a three-arm study comparing radiotherapy, orchiectomy and combined modality treatment using radiotherapy and orchiectomy. A total of 277 patients was randomised (Dearnaley *et al.* 1992; Fellows *et al.* 1992) and results showed a significant lengthening of time for development of metastases in the orchiectomy groups. In addition, there was a gain in local control and survival with approximately a 10% improvement in overall survival in the orchiectomy and radiotherapy group compared with the group treated with radiotherapy alone. This difference failed to reach statistical significance. Unfortunately in this trial radiotherapy was given in an unspecified manner compared with the strict quality control in other trials. Finally the RTOG have performed a further study (Protocol 92–02) in which 1,554 men have been treated with initial androgen suppression and radical radiotherapy and have then been randomised either to stop hormone treatment or to continue for a period of 2 years. Preliminary analyses (Hanks *et al.* 2000; Horwitz *et al.* 2001) have shown significant improvements in local control (94% vs 84%, $p = 0.0001$), biochemical control of disease (79% vs 54%, $p = 0.0001$) and freedom from metastases (89% vs 83%, $p = 0.001$), but no overall improvement in disease-specific survival (92% vs 87%, $p = 0.07$). However, for patients with poorly differentiated disease, there was a statistically significant improvement in both disease-specific and overall survival rates.

In an attempt to identify groups of patients who may benefit from combined modality treatment, the RTOG have undertaken an overview of their radiotherapy studies (Roach *et al.* 2000a) and identified four prognostic groupings. Trials that had included a component of androgen suppression were then analysed (Roach *et al.* 2000b). Results appeared to show a survival benefit for risk group II patients with bulky or T3 disease treated with initial androgen suppression. For group III and IV patients who had a combination of T3, high-grade and node-positive cancers; adjuvant hormonal therapy appeared to give a 20% higher survival rate at 8 years (Table 6.4). An insufficient proportion of group I patients had been treated with hormonal therapy to reach conclusions.

Table 6.4 Prognostic groups and impact of combined modality treatment in patients treated with radiotherapy for prostate cancer: analysis of RTOG trials

| Prognostic group | Description | | Disease-specific survival rate (%) | | | Effects of combined modality treatment |
			5 yr	10 yr	15 yr	
I	T1–T2 Nx	GL2–6	96	86	72	Inadequate patient number to reach conclusion
II	(a) T3 Nx (b) T1–T2 Nx (c) N+	GL2–6 GL7 GL2–6	94	75	61	Improvement of disease-specific survival at 8 years using neoadjuvant androgen suppression
III	(a) T3 Nx (b) T1–T2 Nx (c) N+	GL7 GL8–10 GL7	83	62	39	20% improvement in overall survival at 8 years using long-term (adjuvant) androgen suppression
IV	(a) T3 Nx (b) N+	GL8–10 GL 8–10	64	34	27	

GL, Gleason score.

Conclusion

Although these studies have strongly suggested benefits in disease-related outcomes using either neoadjuvant or adjuvant androgen suppression, significant questions remain to be answered. Toxicities of treatment need to be optimally balanced for an individual. Neoadjuvant androgen deprivation and dose escalation using conformal radiotherapy can both produce improvements in local tumour control and their relative benefits and side effects needs to be assessed. Longer-term androgen deprivation will be likely to result in prolonged or permanent impotence, as well as producing the long-term side effects of androgen deprivation, such as hot flushes, fatigue and impaired exercise tolerance. Some of these effects may be moderated using anti-androgens such as bicalutamide, but these agents have their own toxicity profiles, including gynaecomastia, liver toxicity and gastrointestinal upset, as well as impaired potency. Further studies need to address quality-of-life issues as well as disease-related end-points. There also remains doubt about the contribution of radiotherapy to particularly bulky and high-grade cancers and whether or not these patients might be effectively managed with hormonal treatment alone. This question is currently being addressed in an international study, co-ordinated in the UK by the MRC (Trial Protocol PRO7), in which patients are treated with androgen suppression and are randomised as to whether or not they receive additional radiotherapy. Patients need to be fully informed about the potential risks and benefits of these different treatment approaches and the magnitude of gains that can realistically be expected from combined modality treatment, so that they can make appropriate decisions about their management.

Acknowledgements

This work was undertaken in the Royal Marsden NHS Trust which received a proportion of its funding from the NHS Executive. The views expressed in this publication are those of the authors and not necessarily those of the NHS Executive. This work was supported by the Institute of Cancer Research, the Bob Champion Cancer Trust and the Cancer Research Campaign.

An abbreviated version of this text has been prepared for the Educational Supplement to the ECCO-11 Conference 2001.

References

Amdur RJ, Parsons JT, Fitzgerald LT, Million RR (1990). Adenocarcinoma of the prostate treated with external-beam radiation therapy: 5-year minimum follow-up. *Radiotherapy and Oncology* **18**, 235–246

Aristizabal SA, Steinbronn D, Heusinkveld RS (1984). External beam radiotherapy in cancer of the prostate. *Radiotherapy and Oncology* **1**, 309–315

Beard CJ, Propert KJ, Rieker PP *et al.* (1997) Complications after treatment with external-beam irradiation in early-stage prostate cancer patients: a prospective multiinstitutional outcomes study. *Journal of Clinical Oncology* **15**, 223–229

Bolla M, Gonzalez D, Warde P *et al.* (1997). Improved survival in patients with locally advanced prostate cancer treated with radiotherapy and goserelin [see comments]. *New England Journal of Medicine* **337**, 295–300

Chodak GW, Thisted RA, Gerber GS *et al.* (1994). Results of conservative management of clinically localized prostate cancer. *New England Journal of Medicine* **330**, 242–248

COIN Guidelines (1999). Guidelines on the management of prostate cancer. *Clinical Oncology* **11**, S55–S88

Consensus Conference (1987). The management of clinically localized prostate cancer. *Journal of the American Medical Association* **258**, 2727–2730

Crook J, Robertson S, Collin G, Zaleski V, Esche B (1993). Clinical relevance of trans-rectal ultrasound, biopsy and serum prostate-specific antigen following external beam radiotherapy for carcinoma of the prostate. *International Journal of Radiation Oncology, Biology, Physics* **27**, 31–37

D'Amico AV, Whittington R, Kaplan I *et al.* (1997). Equivalent biochemical failure-free survival after external beam radiation therapy or radical prostatectomy in patients with a pretreatment prostate specific antigen of > 4–20 ng/ml. *International Journal of Radiation Oncology, Biology, Physics* **37**, 1053–1058

De Wit L, Ang KK, van der Schueren E (1983). Acute side effects and late complications after radiotherapy of localized carcinoma of the prostate. *Cancer Treatment Review* **10**, 79–89

Dearnaley DP (2000). Combined modality treatment with radiotherapy and hormonal treatment in localised prostate cancer. In Belldegrun A, Kirby RS, Newling DWW (eds) *New Perspective in Prostate Cancer*, 2nd edn. Oxford: Isis Medical Media, pp 169–180

Dearnaley DP & Melia J (1997). Early prostate cancer – to treat or not to treat. *The Lancet* **349**, 892–893

Dearnaley DP, Horwich A, Shearer RJ (1992). Treatment of advanced localised prostatic cancer by orchidectomy, radiotherapy or combined treatment. A Medical Research Council Study. *British Journal of Urology* **72**, 673–674

Dearnaley DP, Khoo V S, Norman A *et al.* (1999). Comparison of radiation side-effects of conformal and conventional radiotherapy in prostate cancer: a randomised trial. *The Lancet* **353**, 267–272

Duncan W, Warde P, Catton CN (1993). Carcinoma of the prostate: results of radical radiotherapy (1970–1985). *International Journal of Radiation Oncology, Biology, Physics* **26**, 203–210

Fellows GJ, Clark PB, Beynon LL *et al.* (1992). Treatment of advanced localised prostatic cancer by orchiectomy, radiotherapy, or combined treatment. A Medical Research Council Study. *British Journal of Urology* **70**, 304–309

Fiveash J, Hanks G *et al.* (2000). 3D conformal radiation therapy (3DCRT) for the high grade prostate cancer: a multi-institutional review. *International Journal of Radiation Oncology, Biology, Physics* **47**, 335–342

Forman JD, Zinreich E, Lee Ding-Jen, Wharam MD, Baumgardner RA, Order SE (1985). Improving the therapeutic ratio of external beam irradiation for carcinoma of the prostate, *International Journal of Radiation Oncology, Biology, Physics* **11**, 2073–2080

Forman JD, Kumar R, Haas G, Montie J, Porter AT, Mesina CF (1995). Neoadjuvant hormonal downsizing of localised carcinoma of the prostate: effects on the volume of normal tissue irradiation. *Cancer Investigation* **13**, 8–15

Freiha FS, Bagshaw MA (1984). Carcinoma of the prostate: Results of post-irradiation biopsy. *Prostate* **5**, 19–25

Fuks Z, Leibel SA, Wallner KE *et al.* (1991). The effect of local control on metastatic dissemination in carcinoma of the prostate: long-term results in patients treated with 125I implantation. *International Journal of Radiation Oncology, Biology, Physics* **21**, 537–547

Goffinet DR & Bagshaw MA (1990). Radiation therapy of prostate carcinoma: thirty year experience at Stanford University. In Schroder FH (ed.) *EORTC Genitourinary Group Monograph 8. Treatment of Prostatic Cancer – Facts and Controversies*. New York: Wiley-Liss Inc., pp 209–222

Granfors T, Modig H, Damber JE, Tomic R (1998). Combined orchiectomy and external radiotherapy versus radiotherapy alone for nonmetastatic prostate cancer with or without pelvic lymph node involvement: a prospective randomized study. *Journal of Urology* **159**, 2030–2034

Hankey B, Feuer E, Clegg L *et al.* (1999). Cancer surveillance series: interpreting trends in prostate cancer – Part I: Evidence of the effects of screening in recent prostate cancer incidence, mortality, and survival rates. *Journal of the National Cancer Institute* **91**, 1017–1024

Hanks GE, Diamond JJ, Krall JM, Martz KL, Kramer S (1987). A ten year follow-up of 682 patients treated for prostate cancer with radiation therapy in the United States, *International Journal of Radiation Oncology, Biology, Physics* **13**, 499–505

Hanks GE, Krail JM, Martz KL, Diamond JJ, Kramer S (1988a). The outcome of treatment of 313 patients with T-1 (UICC) prostate cancer treated with external beam irradiation. *International Journal of Radiation Oncology, Biology, Physics* **14**, 243–248

Hanks GE, Martz KL, Diamond JJ (1988b). The effect of dose on local control of prostate cancer. *International Journal of Radiation Oncology, Biology, Physics* **15**, 1299–1305

Hanks GE, Hanlon AL, Hudes G, Lee WR, Suasin W, Schultheiss TE (1996a). Patterns-of-failure analysis of patients with high pretreatment prostate-specific antigen levels treated by radiation therapy: the need for improved systemic and locoregional treatment. *Journal of Clinical Oncology* **14**, 1093–1097

Hanks GE, Lee WR, Hanlon AL *et al.* (1996b). Conformal technique dose escalation for prostate cancer: biochemical evidence of improved cancer control with higher doses inpatients with pretreatment prostate-specific antigen > or = 10 ng/ml [see comments]. *International Journal of Radiation Oncology, Biology, Physics* **35**, 861–868

Hanks GE, Hanlon AL, Schultheiss TE (1998). Dose escalation with 3D conformal treatment: five year outcomes, treatment optimisation, and future directions. *International Journal of Radiation Oncology, Biology, Physics* **41**, 501–510

Hanks GE, Lu J, Machtay M *et al.* (2000). RTOG Protocol 92–02. A phase III trial of the use of long term androgen suppression following neoadjuvant cytoreduction and radiotherapy in locally advanced carcinoma of the prostate. *Thirty-sixth Annual Meeting of the American Society of Clinical Oncology* (ASCO), 20–23 May 2000, New Orleans, Louisiana, USA, vol. 19, p 327a (Abstract 1284)

Hanlon A & Hanks G (2000). Failure pattern implications following external beam irradiation of prostate cancer: long-term follow-up and indications of cure. *Cancer Journal of Scientific American* Suppl 2, S193–S197

Horwitz E, Winter K, Hanks G, Lawton C, Russell A, Machtay M (2001). Subset analysis of RTOG 85–31 and 86–10 indicates an advantage for long-term vs. short-term adjuvant hormones for patients with locally advanced nonmetastatic prostate cancer treated with radiation therapy. *International Journal of Radiation Oncology, Biology, Physics* **49**, 947–956

Joon DL, Hasegawa M, Sikes C (1997). Supraadditive apoptotic response of R3327-G rat prostate tumors to androgen ablation and radiation. *International Journal of Radiation Oncology, Biology, Physics* **38**, 1071–1077

Kattan M, Zelefsky M, Kupelian P, Scardino P, Fuks Z, Leibel S (2000). Pretreatment nomogram for predicting the outcome of three-dimensional conformal radiotherapy in prostate cancer. *Journal of Clinical Oncology* **18**, 3352–3359

Laverdiere J, Gomez JL, Cusan L *et al.* (1997). Beneficial effect of combination hormonal therapy administered prior and following external beam radiation therapy in localized prostate cancer. *International Journal of Radiation Oncology, Biology, Physics* **37**, 247–252

Lawton C, Winter K, Murray K *et al.* (2001). Updated results of the Phase III Radiation Therapy Oncology Group (RTOG) Trial 85–31 Evaluating the potential benefit of androgen suppression following standard radiation therapy for unfavorable prognosis carcinoma of the prostate. *International Journal of Radiation Oncology, Biology, Physics* **49**, 937–946

Leibel SA, Hanks GE, Kramer S (1984). Patterns of care outcome studies: Results of the national practice in adenocarcinoma of the prostate. *International Journal of Radiation Oncology, Biology, Physics* **10**, 401–409

Leibel SA, Zelefsky MJ, Kutcher GJ *et al*. (1994). The biological basis and clinical application of 3-dimensional conformal external beam radiation therapy in carcinoma of the prostate. *Seminars in Oncology* **21**, 580–597

Litwin M, Hays R, Fink A *et al*. (1995). Quality-of-life outcomes in men treated for localized prostate cancer. *Journal of the American Medical Association* **273**, 129–135

Lowe BA & Listrom MB (1988). Incidental carcinoma of the prostate: an analysis of the predictors of progression, *Journal of Urology* **140**, 1340–1344

Lu Yao GL & Yao SL (1997). Population-based study of long-term survival in patients with clinically localised prostate cancer [see comments]. *The Lancet* **349**, 906–910

Mithal N & Hoskin P (1990). External beam radiotherapy for carcinoma of the prostate: A retrospective study. *Clinical Oncology* **18**, 297–301

Perez C, William R, Ihde D (1989). Carcinoma of the prostate. In Vincent T, DeVita J, Samuel Hellman, Steven A. Rosenberg (eds) *Cancer: Principle and Practice of Oncology*, Vol. 1, 3rd edn. Philadelphia: JB Lippincott Co., pp 1023–1058

Perez CA, Pilepich MV, Garcia D, Simpson JR, Zivnuska F, Hederman M (1988). Definitive radiation therapy in carcinoma of the prostate localised to the pelvis: Experience at the Mallinckrodt Institute of Radiology. *National Cancer Institute Monographs* **7**, 85–94

Pilepich MV, Krall JM, Sause WT *et al*. (1987). Prognostic factors in carcinoma of the prostate-analysis of RTOG study 7506. *International Journal of Radiation Oncology, Biology, Physics* **13**, 339–349

Pilepich MV, Krall JM, al Sarraf M *et al*. (1995). Androgen deprivation with radiation therapy compared with radiation therapy alone for locally advanced prostatic carcinoma: a randomized comparative trial of the Radiation Therapy Oncology Group. *Urology* **45**, 616–623

Pilepich MV, Caplan R, Byhardt RW *et al*. (1997). Phase III trial of androgen suppression using goserelin in unfavorable- prognosis carcinoma of the prostate treated with definitive radiotherapy: Report of Radiation Therapy Oncology Group protocol 85–31. *Journal of Clinical Oncology* **15**, 1013–1021

Pilepich MV, Winter K, Roach M *et al*. (1998). Phase III Radiation Oncology Group (RTOG) 86–10 of androgen deprivation before and during radiotherapy in locally advanced carcinoma of the prostate. *Proceedings of the American Society of Clinical Oncology* **17**, 308a (Abstract 1185)

Pollack A, Zaggars G, Smith L *et al*. (2000). Preliminary results of a randomized radiotherapy dose-escalation study comparing 70 Gy with 78 Gy for prostate cancer. *Journal of Clinical Oncology* **18**, 3904–3911

Porter A, Ethliali M, Manji MEA (1998). A phase III randomised trial to evaluate the efficacy of neoadjuvant therapy prior to curative radiotherapy in locally advanced prostate cancer patients. A Canadian Urologic Oncology Group study. *Proceedings of the American Society of Clinical Oncology* **17**, 315a (Abstract 1123)

Potosky A, Legler J, Albertsen P *et al*. (2000). Health outcomes after prostatectomy or radiotherapy for prostate cancer: results from the Prostate Cancer Outcomes Study. *Journal of the National Cancer Institute* **92**, 1582–1592

Roach MI, Chinn DM, Holland J, Clarke M (1996). A pilot survey of sexual function and quality of life following 3D conformal radiotherapy for clinically localised prostate cancer. *International Journal of Radiation Oncology, Biology, Physics* **35**, 869–874

Roach M III, Lu J, Pilepich M *et al.* (2000a). Four prognostic groups predict long-term survival from prostate cancer following radiotherapy alone on radiation therapy oncology group clinical trials. *International Journal of Radiation Oncology, Biology, Physics* **47**, 609–615

Roach M III, Lu J, Pilepich M *et al.* (2000b). Predicting long-term survival, and the need for hormonal therapy: a meta-analysis of RTOG prostate cancer trials. *International Journal of Radiation Oncology, Biology, Physics* **47**, 617–627

Sagerman RH, Chun HC, King GA, Chung CT, Dalal PS (1989). External beam radiotherapy for carcinoma of the prostate. *Cancer* **63**, 2468–2474

Sandler HM, Perez-Tamayo C, Ten Haken RK, Lichter AS (1992) Dose escalation for stage C(T3) prostate cancer: minimal rectal toxicity observed using conformal therapy. *Radiotherapy and Oncology* **23**, 53–54

Scardino PT & Bretas F (1987). Interstitial radiotherapy. In Bruce AW, Trachtenberg J (eds) *Adenocarcinoma of the Prostate*. London: Springer-Verlag, pp 145–158

Seddon B, Bidmead M, Wilson J, Khoo V, Dearnaley D (2000). Target volume definition in conformal radiotherapy for prostate cancer: quality assurance in the MRC RT-01 trial. *Radiotherapy and Oncology* **56**, 73–83

Shearer RJ, Davies JH, Gelister JSK, Dearnaley DP (1992). Hormonal cytoreduction and radiotherapy for carcinoma of the prostate. *British Journal of Urology* **69**, 521–524

Shipley W, Thames H, Sandler H *et al.* (1999). Radiation therapy for clinically localized prostate cancer: a multi-institutional pooled analysis. *Journal of the American Medical Association* **281**, 1598–1604

Valicenti R, Lu J, Pilepich M, Asbell S, Grignon D (2000). Survival advantage from higher-dose radiation therapy for clinically localized prostate cancer treated on the Radiation Therapy Oncology Group trials. *Journal of Clinical Oncology* **18**, 2740–2746

Vicini F, Kestin L, Martinez A (2000). The correlation of serial prostate specific antigen measurements with clinical outcome after external beam radiation therapy of patients for prostate carcinoma. *Cancer* **88**, 2305–2318

Widmark A, Fransson P, Tavelin B (1994). Self-assessment questionnaire for evaluating urinary and intestinal late side effects after pelvic radiotherapy in patients with prostate cancer compared with an age-matched control population. *Cancer* **74**, 2520–2532

Yorke ED, Fuks Z, Norton L, Whitmore W, Ling CC (1993). Modeling the development of metastasis from primary and locally recurrent tumours: Comparison with a clinical data base for prostatic cancer. *Cancer Research* **53**, 2987–2993

Zagars GK, von Eschenback AC, Johnson DE, Oswald MJ (1987). Stage C adenocarcinoma of the prostate: An analysis of 551 patients treated with external beam radiation. *Cancer* **60**, 1489–1499

Zelefsky MJ, Leibel SA, Burman CM *et al.* (1994). Neoadjuvant hormonal therapy improves the therapeutic ratio in patients with bulky prostatic cancer treated with three-dimensional conformal radiation therapy. *International Journal of Radiation Oncology, Biology, Physics* 755–761

Zelefsky M, Leibel S, Gaudin P *et al.* (1998). Dose escalation with three-dimensional conformal radiation therapy affects the outcome in prostate cancer. *International Journal of Radiation Oncology, Biology, Physics* **41**, 491–500

Zelefsky M, Cowen D, Fuks Z *et al.* (1999). Long term tolerance of high dose three-dimensional conformal radiotherapy in patients with localized prostate carcinoma. *Cancer* **85**, 2460–2468

Zelefsky M, Fuks Z, Happersett L *et al.* (2000). Clinical experience with intensity modulated radiation therapy (IMRT) in prostate cancer. *Radiotherapy and Oncology* **55**, 241–249

Zietman AL, Shipley WU, Willett GC (1993). Residual disease after radical surgery or radiation therapy for prostate cancer. Clinical significance and therapeutic implications. *Cancer* **71**, 859–869

Zietman AL, Prince EA, Nakfoor BM, Park JJ (1997). Androgen deprivation and radiation therapy: sequencing studies using the Shionogi in vivo tumor system. *International Journal of Radiation Oncology, Biology, Physics* **38**, 1067–1070

Chapter 7

The clinical utility of brachytherapy for localised prostate cancer

Dan Ash

Introduction

If the aim of radiotherapy is to deliver as high a dose as possible to the smallest possible volume while sparing adjacent normal tissue, then brachytherapy is the best way of achieving this and constitutes the ultimate conformal therapy. It is also possible to modulate the intensity of the radiation to increase the radiation dose to known areas of tumour, while sparing critical normal structures such as the urethra and the rectum.

Modern ultrasonography and template-guided brachytherapy for localised prostate cancer have been practised for the last 15 years and there are now several hundred patients reported in the literature with more than 5 years of follow-up (Blasko *et al.* 1995; Stock *et al.* 1996; Beyer & Priestley 1997; Zelefsky *et al.* 2000). There are, however, very few patients for whom 10-year follow-up data are available (Ragde *et al.* 1998).

Although there are no randomised controlled clinical trials to confirm the superiority of any form of radical local treatment for prostate cancer in comparison with any other, there is enough information to identify those patients who are likely to do well with brachytherapy and the key factors of technique and implant quality that will achieve consistently good results.

Patient selection

There are two aspects to patient selection: one is to define patients who are likely to have a good outcome in terms of biochemical disease-free survival and the other is to identify patients who will have a good functional outcome. For the first, the important prognostic factors are presenting prostate-specific antigen (PSA), Gleason score and stage. For functional outcome the most important factor is the state of the urinary outflow. This is best described by the International Prostate Symptom Score and by the prostate volume.

It is possible to define three prognostic groups:

1. Good: PSA <10, Gleason score ≤6.
2. Intermediate: PSA 10–20, ± Gleason score 7.
3. Poor: PSA >20 + Gleason score >7.

Investigations

For patients treated by brachytherapy alone, tumour should be confined within the prostate capsule without evidence of spread outside. Patients should therefore have the following investigations: PSA; transrectal ultrasonography to measure prostate volume and assess extent of disease; biopsy-proven adenocarcinoma with Gleason score; computed tomography (CT) or magnetic resonance imaging (MRI) to stage pelvic nodes; dedicated pelvic MRI to assess local extent of disease; and bone scan in patients who have a PSA >10.

Indications

Patients should have a life expectancy of greater than 5 years. Their disease should be confined within the prostate capsule. There should be no evidence of metastases. The prostate volume should be less than 50 cm^3 and the PSA should be less than 30.

Contraindications

Patients who have had a recent transurethral resection of the prostate (TURP) with a large prostatic cavity are not suitable for brachytherapy, both because it is difficult to position seeds within the prostate and because there is a significant risk of urethral morbidity leading to incontinence (Grimm et al. 1997).

For patients with presenting gland volumes of more than 50 cm^3 there is a higher risk of side effects and complications, and there is also a high probability that some of the prostate will not be accessible to seed implantation because it has grown behind the pubic arch. For these patients, 3 months of neoadjuvant hormone therapy will reduce prostate volume by approximately 30% and shrink the prostate volume down to less than 50 cm^3 for many of them (Blasko et al. 1993).

Patients in the good prognosis group have a high probability of biochemical disease-free control with brachytherapy alone and will have good functional outcomes if the prostate is less than 40 cm^3 with minimal lower urinary tract symptoms before treatment.

For the intermediate groups it has been suggested that outcomes might be improved by adding external beam radiation to brachytherapy and by giving adjuvant hormone therapy. At present there is insufficient evidence to confirm that these measures are beneficial. For the poor prognostic group, local treatment alone is unlikely to be sufficient because these patients have a high probability of occult metastatic disease.

Technique

The key to consistent implant quality is image-guided source placement which is usually performed with interactive real-time ultrasonography. Needle placement is also guided by a template, the co-ordinates of which are transmitted over the ultrasonic image (Grimm et al. 1994).

Pre-planning

Before performing the implant it is helpful to have an accurate measurement of prostate volume and to produce a dose and seed plan from a transrectal ultrasonographic volume study. Ultrasound sections of 5 mm are taken from prostate base to apex with the template co-ordinates displayed on each section. These data can be used to calculate the exact number and position of seeds required for the implant. It is usual to deliver more seeds to the periphery of the prostate than the centre, in order to avoid excessive doses to the urethra.

It is now possible to combine the pre-plan with the implant under the same anaesthetic so that repositioning of the patient between the two phases is avoided.

Dose prescription

For permanent iodine-125 seed implants the usual dose for patients who receive brachytherapy alone is 145 Gy. This is the minimum dose delivered to the prostate capsule plus a margin of 2–3 mm. Approximately 50% of the prostate volume may receive 50% or more than that dose. The urethral dose is kept below 200 Gy wherever possible. When iodine seed implantation is used as a boost after 45–50 Gy external beam radiation, the dose is reduced to 110 Gy (Prestidge *et al.* 1998).

For patients treated with paladium seed implants, the total dose is reduced to account for the more rapid dose rate (iodine-125 half-life is 59.4 days, paladium-103 half-life 17 days). The dose is therefore 115 Gy for patients treated by brachytherapy alone and 90 Gy when it is combined with external beam radiation.

Removable implants are mostly given with high-dose rate radiation after external beam radiation and are delivered in two to four fractions of 5–15 Gy.

Post-implant dosimetry

For surgery, one of the key quality indices is the status of the resection margin. Similarly, for brachytherapy, confirmation that the target volume has been adequately covered to an adequate dose is strongly correlated with outcome.

Post-implant dosimetry is most usually done with a CT scan 4–6 weeks after implantation. This enables the prostate volume and the position of the seeds to be re-entered into a computer planning programme. The key quality index shown to be related to outcome is the D90, which is the dose received by 90% of the target volume. If this is 90% or more than the prescribed dose, the probability of biochemical control is very high and, conversely, failure to achieve a satisfactory D90 is associated with a higher probability of biochemical relapse (Stock *et al.* 1998).

Side effects and complications

Nearly all patients develop a variable degree of urethritis after brachytherapy. This usually starts 4 or 5 days after the implant and may last for 2–3 weeks. These symptoms then settle but frequency, urgency and nocturia may take 4 or 5 months to settle gradually. Only 2–3% of patients still have significant urinary symptoms at 1 year (Gelblum *et al.* 1999).

The risk of incontinence is approximately 1% but can be much higher in patients who have had a previous TURP, particularly if this is within a few months of brachytherapy (Grimm *et al.* 1997).

It is usual to cover the implant with antibiotics and infection and bleeding in the acute phase are rare events. However, 12–15% of patients may develop acute retention. The risk is higher in patients who have significant lower urinary tract symptoms and enlarged prostates before brachytherapy (Terk *et al.* 1998).

A few patients may have temporary proctitis. The risk of serious rectal injury such as fistula is 0.1–0.2%.

Brachytherapy may cause impotence in approximately one-third of treated patients. The risk is higher in men aged over 70 and in those in whom there is already some erectile dysfunction (Arterbery *et al.* 1997). Of patients who develop impotence after brachytherapy, 80–90% have potency restored by sildenafil (Viagra).

Results

The key outcome measures are overall survival, freedom from clinical progression, local control and biochemical disease-free survival. Although it is imperfect and cannot distinguish local from distant relapse, post-treatment PSA is currently considered the most sensitive and objective outcome measure by which to evaluate prostate cancer treatments. Biochemical failure is defined as three successive rises in PSA with at least 3 months between each. Biochemical control is defined by the achievement of a certain PSA nadir. Most reports use a PSA level of less than 1 to define biochemical control, but some suggest that this should be 0.5. Unlike surgery, the PSA does not fall to zero after radiation and the nadir may not be achieved for 12–18 months.

For good-prognosis patients treated by brachytherapy alone, approximately 80% are biochemically controlled at 5 years and approximately 70% at 10 years (Stock *et al.* 1996; Grimm *et al.* 1997).

The incidence of clinical failure is, however, much less because this may not occur until 3–5 years after biochemical failure.

For intermediate-prognosis patients, biochemical control is achieved in 40–50% of cases. For poor-prognosis patients, control is only achieved in 20–30%.

Comparison with other treatments

Unfortunately there are no randomised controlled clinical trials that compare any radical local treatment with any other or with the no-treatment option. The comparisons that have been made are confounded by different case selection, different case mix, different length of follow-up and inadequate information on the quality of the treatment delivered.

Matched-pair analysis for good prognosis patients treated by either radical prostatectomy or brachytherapy has shown very similar outcomes (Ramos *et al.* 1999). The general message is that good prognosis patients do better than poor ones, however treated.

Management of PSA failure

Patients who develop an isolated PSA failure without disease outside the prostate are theoretically eligible for radical salvage treatment by surgery. This is, however, a high-risk option (Tefilli *et al.* 1998). It is not possible to give radical external beam radiation after brachytherapy and the mainstay of salvage treatment is therefore hormone therapy which cannot be considered curative. For many patients with very slowly rising PSA at low level, it is reasonable to maintain them on surveillance before starting hormone treatment.

Conclusion

In spite of the absence of randomised clinical trials, there is considerable experience from several hundred patients, which demonstrates that good-prognosis localised prostate cancer treated by brachytherapy alone is associated with a high probability of biochemical disease-free control with a low risk of side effects and complications. The treatment is, however, technically demanding and is best performed by dedicated teams in large centres with a sufficient caseload to maintain high levels of expertise.

References

Arterbery VE, Frazier A, Dalmia P *et al.* (1997). Quality of life after permanent prostate implant. *Seminars in Surgical Oncology* **13**, 461–464

Beyer DC & Priestley JB Jr (1997). Biochemical disease-free survival following 125I prostate implantation. *International Journal of Radiation Oncology* **37**, 1035

Blasko JC, Grimm PD, Radge H (1993). Brachytherapy and organ preservation in the management of carcinoma of the prostate. *Seminars in Radiation Oncology* **3**, 240–249

Blasko JC, Wallner K Grimmm PD *et al.* (1995). Prostate specific antigen based disease control following ultrasound guided ^{125}iodine implantation for stage T1/T2 prostatic carcinoma. *Journal of Urology* 1096–1099

Gelblum DY, Potters L, Ashley R *et al.* (1999). Urinary morbidity following ultrasound guided transperineal prostate seed implantation. *Radiation Oncology Biology Physics* **45**, 59–67

Grimm PD, Blasko JC, Ragde H (1994). Ultrasound guided transperineal implantation of iodine-125 and palladium-103 for the treatment of early stage prostate cancer – technical concepts in planning, operative technique and evaluation. *Atlas of the Urology Clinics North America* **2**, 113–125

Grimm P, Blasko J, Ragde H *et al.* (1997). Transperineal ultrasound guided I-125/Pd-103 brachytherapy in the management of localised prostate cancer: Update of the clinical experience at seven years (Abstr). *International Journal of Radiation Oncology Biology Physics* **39**, 219

Prestidge BR, Bice WS, Kiefer EJ *et al.* (1998). Timing of computed tomography-based postimplant assessment following permanent transperineal prostate brachytherapy. *International Journal of Radiation Oncology Biology Physics* **40**, 1111–1115

Ragde H, El Gamal AA, Snow PB *et al.* (1998). Ten year disease free survival after transperineal sonography guided iodine-125 brachytherapy with or without 45 Gy external beam irradiation in the treatment of prostates with clinically localised low to high Gleason grade prostate carcinoma.*Cancer* **83**, 989–1001

Ramos CG, Carvalhal GF, Smith DS *et al.* (1999). Retrospective comparison of radical retropubic prostatectomy and Iodine 125 brachytherapy for localised prostate cancer. *Journal of Urology* **161**, 1212–1215

Stock RG, Stone NN, DeWyngaert JK *et al.* (1996). Prostate specific antigen findings and biopsy results following interactive ultrasound guided transperineal brachytherapy for early stage prostate carcinoma. *Cancer* **77**, 2386–2392

Stock RG, Stone NN, Tabert A *et al.* (1998). A dose-response study for iodine 125 prostate implants. *International Journal of Radiation Oncology Biology Physics* **41**, 101–108

Tefilli MV, Gheiler EL, Tiguert R *et al.* (1998). Salvage surgery or salvage radiotherapy for locally recurrent prostate cancer. *Urology* 224–229

Terk MD, Stock RG, Stone NN (1998). Identification of patients at increased risk for prolonged urinary retention following radioactive seed implantation of the prostate. *Journal of Urology* **160**, 1379–1382

Zelefsky MJ, Hollister T, Raben A *et al.* (2000). Five year biochemical outcome and toxicity with transperineal CT-planned permanent 125I prostate implantation for patients with localised prostate cancer. *International Journal of Radiation Oncology Biology Physics* **47**, 1261–1266

Medical interventions relevant in prevention and management of early prostate cancer: a new potential role for GPs, schools' and works' medical officers, as well as STD, family planning and infertility clinics

R Tim D Oliver, Tim Lane, Paula Wells, Frank Chinegwundoh and Vinod Nargund

Introduction

The only randomised trial to investigate the role of active intervention in early prostate cancer was grossly underpowered (Iversen *et al*. 1995). As a result today it is increasingly important to respond to patient choice (Auvinen 2001). As a consequence there continues to be considerable debate on the value of radical prostatectomy or radiation (Kuban *et al*. 2000) compared with expected treatment (Albertson 2000) in the management of early prostate cancer. What few large-scale phase II data there are (Chodak & Palmer 1996) suggest that only the small minority with the most malignant high-grade tumours obtain significant benefit. However, as such cases are often highly metastatic, selection by screening to exclude TMN classification N+ and M+ cases could be a major factor in the apparent gain from early intervention in this subgroup of patients. This lack of unequivocal proof of gain from early intervention is the most significant factor that fuels the uncertainty of those who reserve judgement on the benefits of prostate-specific antigen (PSA) screening.

There is no doubt that detection of PSA above 10 predicts probability of mortality from prostate cancer (Parkes *et al*. 1995), and that in populations such as in the USA where screening for PSA is widespread, there is a marked stage shift with reduction in incidence of patients with M+ disease at presentation (Mettlin *et al*. 1998). This means that surgeons in the USA, by primarily selecting patients with PSA < 10 for surgery have the greatest possibility of operating on potentially curable patients, and that their results bear no comparison with those at the time the only randomised trial of surgical intervention was attempted. However, such a selection will also increase the number who may not need treatment.

Until recently there has been little discussion of the potential for medical intervention in management of early prostate cancer. The recent reports that dietary selenium (Clark *et al*. 1996), lycopene (Giovannucci *et al*. 1995) and fat (Hayes *et al*. 1999; Meyer *et al*. 1999), as well as solar-induced vitamin D (Hanchette & Schwartz

1992; Corder *et al.* 1993; Luscombe *et al.* 2001), may play a role in influencing prostate cancer risk are beginning to provide a justification for increased interest in the role of nutrition in prostate cancer development, and the potential for gain from encouraging changes in diet as part of medical intervention. Possible additional support for this view comes from reports that dietary intervention in advanced cases favourably changes parameters of disease activity (Schmitz-Drager *et al.* 2001). Further evidence of the benefit of influencing host resistance comes from postmortem studies, which demonstrate that 30% of men aged over 40 have prostatic intraepithelial neoplasia (Sakr *et al.* 1995), whereas in the absence of screening fewer than 1 in 20 die of prostate cancer at the peak age of death, i.e. 70–75 years. Such observations, and the fact that initial age of onset of sexual activity and testosterone levels at the time of puberty are important factors in prostate cancer initiation (Ross *et al.* 1992; Key 1995), provide a clear indication that risk factors involved in development of prostate cancer from prostatic intraepithelial neoplasia to lethal cancer act over a long period.

One possible common pathway hypothesised to explain these facts and how they link with the physical risk factors associated with prostate cancer, such as immunosuppressive pesticides (Bekesi *et al.* 1983; Fleming *et al.* 1999) and radiation (Beral *et al.* 1985), is that there is increased vulnerability of the growing peripubertal prostate to lifetime persistence of subclinical 'honeymoon' prostatitis (Oliver 1995, 2000; Oliver *et al.* 2001). Possible evidence to support this hypothesis is that prostate cancer mortality has begun to fall in both the UK and the USA at the same time, despite widely differing policies on PSA screening (Oliver *et al.* 2000b). Even in the USA it is difficult to accept that screening is a major factor in the decline because it penetrates only to the richer half of the population. In addition, as it leads to diagnosis of cancer in men 10 years younger than would be dying from it in the absence of post-screen-detected surgery, screening would not be expected to have such an immediate effect (particularly as PSA screening undoubtedly contributed to part of the much greater increase in incidence in the 1990s). Mortality began to decline within 1–2 years of screening being introduced into the USA. A similar decline also occurred in the UK in the absence of screening (Table 8.1). It certainly could be that part of the reduced mortality comes from the increased use of hormone therapy to treat patients found through screening to have M+ disease. However, an additional factor that is

Table 8.1 Annual percentage change in prostate cancer incidence and mortality

	USA		UK	
	Incidence (%)	Mortality rate (%)	Incidence (%)	Mortality rate (%)
1985–89	+6.9	+0.7	+1.8	+0.6
1989–91	+18	+3.1	+2.3	+0.5
1991–95	−12.8	−1.9	+2.5	+0.3
1995–98	NA	−7	−6.2	−0.5

common in both the USA and the UK is the fact that, 10–15 years before the decline occurred, there was widespread increased use of safe sex in response to the HIV epidemic which was associated with a major reduction of sexually transmitted disease (STD) (particularly gonorrhoea) and presumably also coincident subclinical prostatitis (Table 8.2). A similar decline in prostate cancer was noted in 1960 which was linked to a previous decline in gonorrhoea (Heshmat et al. 1975).

Given the 6- to 8-year lead time predictive power of PSA elevation to identify patients at risk of prostate cancer death (Parkes 1995), it would be interesting to know whether there has been a decline of serum PSA in population-based serum banks that predates the recent mortality decline, although it still post-dates the AIDS 'Safe Sex Campaign'.

Table 8.2 UK prostate cancer mortality and incidence compared with STD incidence and condom sales

	1950–55	1975	1986	1990	1995	1998
Gonorrhoea	16,000	60,000	48,000	10,000	9,000	12,393
Condom sales (UK)	NA	NA	138 × 106	NA	NA	160 × 106
Cancer of the prostate						
Incidence (%)	NA	32.9	46.6	53.4	65.6	56.1
Mortality rate (%)	15.6	19.1	24.7	27.0	29.6	27.4

These observations suggest that simple short-term public health interventions might be having as marked an effect in early stages of the disease as those being achieved from the use of tamoxifen in women at high risk of breast cancer (Anonymous 1998). Taken with recent reports of the use of better tolerated androgen-blocking drugs, such as bicalutamide (Casodex), in early prostate cancer in some instances without surgery or radiation (Abrahamsson 2001; See et al. 2001), these observations provide an early indication of the potential of focusing medical intervention as part of a broader strategy in management of early prostate cancer and its prevention. This chapter aims to review these data and to explore the potential of medical treatment to complement surgery and radiation in the management of early prostate cancer.

Relevance of modern epidemiology to potential of medical intervention in treatment of early prostate cancer

There are an increasing number of clinical situations where a link has been established between subclinical infection and malignant progression of cancer (Danesh et al. 1997). The oldest is the linkage between chronic osteomyelitis and osteogenic sarcoma (Petrikowski et al. 1995). In the 1980s a link, albeit indirect, was demonstrated between hepatoma and consumption of the hepatotoxic substance aflatoxin produced by fungal contamination of groundnuts (Ross *et al.* 1992). The 1990s have seen an increasing acceptance of the link between persistent gastric infection with *Helicobacter pylori* and stomach cancer (Forman 1996), which is thought to be mediated by inflammatory cytokine-induced proliferation of gastric mucosa (Crabtree *et al.* 1994).

It is now 6 years since the first speculation that subclinical prostatitis might be playing a similar role in the development of prostate cancer (Oliver *et al.* 1995). This was done on the basis of two epidemiological data sets: first, the geographical epidemiology of latent versus invasive prostate cancer (Breslow *et al.* 1977; Oishi *et al.* 1995) and how it closely matched that of cervix and penile cancer as well as heterosexual acquired immune deficient syndrome (AIDS). The second was an overview of published prostate cancer epidemiological studies which provided evidence that deficiency of vitamins A and D and high levels of animal fat in the diet increased its risk (Key 1995), as did early age of onset of sexual intercourse and multiple non-specific sexual infections and vasectomy (Table 8.3), possibly related to reduced use of condoms. This was in the early days of vasectomy because the influence has disappeared from most recent studies in the post-HIV era.

Table 8.3 Meta-analysis of epidemiology studies of dietary and sexual behaviour risk factors for prostate cancer (Key 1995)

Behaviour	Relative risk
Animal fat consumption	1.54
Carrot consumption	0.66
Green vegetable consumption	0.93
Early age of first intercourse	1.31
Numbers of sexual partners	1.21
Sexually acquired infection	1.86
Vasectomy	1.54

As it was known that latent prostate cancer was present in a similar frequency worldwide (Breslow *et al.* 1977), it was suggested that these lesions progressed to invasive cancer only as a result of persistent subclinical prostatitis from multiple STDs that were known to be more prevalent (Gerbase *et al.* 1998) in the areas with high risk of invasive prostate cancer. Persistence of infection was favoured by vitamin A deficiency reducing T-cell immunity (Semba *et al.* 1993) and vitamin D deficiency reducing macrophage function (Davies 1995), compounded by the immunosuppressive effect of high pesticide intake (Bekesi *et al.* 1983; Fleming *et al.* 1999) as a result of their concentration in animal fat. Reports that regular exercise at the time of puberty reduces prostate cancer (Oliveria *et al.* 1996), as it also reduces cancer of the testes, breast and colon, may also be explained in part by the prostatitis hypothesis because in women regular exercise before puberty delays its onset. If this occurred, in men, it would reduce risk of early underage STDs (Brabin 2001).

Genital hygiene and its relevance to the prostatitis hypothesis

Similar to heterosexual transmission of HIV infection, there is increasing evidence that deaths from prostate, cervix and penile cancer are low in areas of the world with high rates of circumcision. It is unclear whether it is circumcision itself that is the cause because these societies in the Middle East also have pubertal ceremonies providing both sexes with education about sexual hygiene. The relative lower incidence in Asian countries where circumcision is not routine is thought to be the result of genes reducing 5α-reductase production because they reduce transformation of testosterone to the intraprostatic active androgen which reduces prostate cancer risk (Ross *et al.* 1992a). An additional factor in Japan is that the main form of contraception is the condom (Warming 1986), which may also contribute to a risk reduction. In India, prostate cancer is less frequent in circumcised Muslims and highest in Hindus (Yeole & Jussawalla 1997) as is cervix and penile cancer (Gajalakshmi & Shanta 1993). This last study also demonstrated that there is an inverse relationship between education and risks of cervix and penile cancer in Hindus (Gajalakshmi & Shanta 1993). The final piece of evidence supporting the hypothesis is the demonstration in African–Americans that circumcision reduces the risk (Ross *et al.* 1987), whereas in Japanese men phimosis and prostatitis (Nakata *et al.* 1993) increase the risk (Table 8.4).

Table 8.4 Risk factors for prostate cancer in Japanese Gunma Prefecture (Nakata *et al.* 1993)

Risk factor	No. at risk	Percentage exposed	Age-adjusted odds ratio
High meat intake			
Prostate cancer	202	15	1.26
Controls	209	12.9	
Low intake of vegetables			
Prostate cancer	125	12	2.89
Controls	112	4.5	
Prostatitis			
Prostate cancer	294	26	4.46
Controls	294	7	
Phimosis			
Prostate cancer	245	34	1.62
Controls	260	24	

Early sexual activity as a cause of prostatitis and its relevance to prostate cancer risk

It has long been known that early onset of sexual intercourse is one of the most important risk factors for the development of cervical cancer (Rotkin 1967). There is now increasing evidence that this risk factor also considerably increases the risk of HIV infection and, as Table 8.3 demonstrates, is a consistent, albeit low-level, risk factor for prostate cancer (Key 1995). For a disease whose most lethal manifestation under normal circumstances only peaks between the ages of 70 and 75, it is difficult to know how responses to epidemiological questionnaires would be reliable in respect of this question, let alone, if it was true, how it could take such a long time to manifest its effect. Recently there have been reports from community-based studies that the cumulative lifetime risk of prostatitis may effect up to 40% of the population (Roberts *et al.* 1998), with its incidence peaking between the ages of 40 and 50.

With reports from postmortem studies (Sakr *et al.* 1995) demonstrating that, between the ages of 40 and 50, up to 20% of men first demonstrate evidence of prostatic intraepithelial neoplasia (Table 8.5), there is clearly a need to focus more attention on an earlier age to understand the factors that initiate prostate cancer. Evidence to support this view comes from a seroepidemiological study which we have undertaken on attendees at an STD clinic that services two gold mines in the town of Carltonville, Gauteng province, South Africa (Oliver *et al.* 2001). Serum originally taken from any attendee for routine screening purposes as part of other prospective research studies was also tested for PSA as a surrogate marker of prostate damage. A total of 343 samples (median age 30 range 18–50) were tested. A subset of 83 of these were interviewed using a standardised questionnaire to establish circumcision status, STD history and previous sexual history.

Table 8.5 Prostate intraepithelial neoplasia (PIN) at postmortem examination in male accident victims (Sakr *et al.* 1995)

Age at postmortem examination (years)	Incidence of PIN (%)	Incidence of cancer (%)
20–29	0	0
30–39	9	0
40–49	20	27
50–59	44	34

In the initial study, 262 sera were tested and there was a statistically significant correlation ($\chi^2 = 4.85$, $p < 0.02$) between level of anti-chlamydial antibody response and level of PSA, in that 37% of 61 patients with high titre ($\geq$ 1 in 64) had a PSA $\geq$ 0.8 whereas the frequency was 17% in 201 samples with low or negative anti-chlamydial antibody titre. Although it is well accepted that serological studies are less certain predictors of chlamydial involvement than antigen-based assays, the invasive nature of the latter requires some degree of validation before they can be justified in a research setting. These preliminary data certainly provide that degree of justification.

A second observation that emerged from this study was that, in the subgroup who participated in the standardised questionnaire, there was a non-significant trend for higher PSA levels in those initiating sex before the age of 16 and in those having more than 20 partners. Surprisingly there was a negative interaction between the two risk factors in that in those who began sex before the age of 16, increasing numbers of sexual partners increased the risk of the individual having an elevated PSA whereas those over 16 years of age had a decreased incidence of raised PSA with increasing number of sexual partners. Although the numbers are too small for definitive conclusions and it could just be a chance observation, there is a possible explanation that would justify further expansion to achieve sufficient numbers to prove or disprove the observation. If early post-puberty infection were associated with poverty and poor nutrition, it would be likely to increase the chance of a Th2 type of enhancing immune response and greater damage from a given level of infection (O'Byrne *et al.* 2000). In contrast late onset of regular sexual activity might ensure a more effective Th1 type of response that eliminated infection more efficiently and the enhanced immune response ensured less prostatic damage despite multiple partners.

These observations provide the justification for population-based school sex education programmes about STDs to be linked to prostate and cervix cancer prevention.

Potential of endocrine treatment to enhance outcomes from conventional treatment of localised prostate cancer

With more than 1,000 patients incorporated into trials of neoadjuvant hormone therapy before radical prostatectomy (Table 8.6), there is absolutely no doubt that such treatment reduces the incidence of tumour in the margins of the operated specimen (Gleave *et al.* 2000). Despite this (albeit with only 5 years of follow-up), the evidence for the impact of this treatment on PSA relapse-free survival is still far from clear. This is in contrast to the smaller numbers entered in trials of hormone therapy before radiation, where three of three trials have a positive outcome in terms of overall survival (Bolla *et al.* 1997; Pilepich *et al.* 1997; Granfors *et al.* 1998). As only two of three have a significant effect on PSA relapse-free survival and there is evidence of a delayed effect of scatter from prostate radiation affecting Leydig cell function, at least part of the benefit may not come from the synergy between endocrine treatment and radiation demonstrated in animal models (Zietman *et al.* 1997).

In contrast to the difficulty of demonstrating survival advantage from neoadjuvant hormone therapy before surgery, hormone therapy given in the adjuvant setting after surgery provides the only positive evidence for improved survival from an interaction between endocrine therapy and surgery. The benefit was demonstrated in patients found to be node positive at the time of surgery (Messing *et al.* 1999). As yet there

Table 8.6 Impact of neoadjuvant hormone therapy on pathological stages at radical prostatectomy (Gleave 2000)

	Control[a]	Three months[a] of hormones	Eight months[b] of hormones
No cancer at surgery (%)	1[c]	2[c]	13
Negative margins (%)	53	78	79
Positive margins (%)	46	20	8

[a]1,420 in seven randomised studies.
[b]156 in a phase II study.
[c]Median value in seven studies.

are no studies to demonstrate whether there is any benefit from combining hormones with interstitial radiation, although this is an increasing pattern of treatment as the results for the external beam studies become more widely disseminated.

Despite the ongoing debates on timing of endocrine interaction with both surgical and radiotherapeutic local treatment of prostate cancer, there is increasing acceptance of the view that endocrine therapy has an even more important role in early disease patients than previously accepted (Kirk 1996). This comes from the immediate versus deferred studies where there is evidence that the benefit from early treatment is more marked for patients with localised than for those with metastatic disease. However, these patients will also be less tolerant of side effects of treatment because they are less frequently symptomatic at the time of diagnosis. With time, these patients end up dying more frequently from non-prostate cancer-related causes, thus nullifying the benefit of early treatment. Furthermore, because of the increased duration of treatment, they are more likely to suffer from delayed late effects such as anaemia (Strum *et al.* 1997) and loss of bone mineral density (Wei *et al.* 1999).

There is one important issue that has emerged from studies of hormone therapy in local disease studies. This is the fact that, in all except one of the trials demonstrating benefit from adding hormones to local therapy, either surgery or radiation, none had an endocrine alone arm (Table 8.7). The only three-arm trial was prematurely stopped because of slow recruitment and it was therefore grossly underpowered. However, in that study, endocrine treatment alone produced a statistically significantly better survival than localised radiation alone, whereas the combination of radiation with endocrine treatment (though significantly better than radiation alone) was no different to hormone therapy alone (Fellow & Clarke 1992).

The case for intermittent rather than continuous endocrine treatment in early as well as metastatic prostate cancer

It has long been recognised that chronic exposure to antibiotics is the best way to induce antibiotic resistance in bacteria. Until recently continuous androgen deprivation has been routine in prostate cancer, in part because of the ease of management after

Table 8.7 Integration of hormones and local therapy in management of M0 prostate cancer

	Radiation or surgery alone (%)	Hormones + radiation surgery (%)	Hormones alone (%)
Pilepich et al. (1995)[a] (4 months ± radiation)	23 (n = 200)	50 (n = 196)	NA
Bolle et al. (1997)[a] (3 years ± radiation)	61 (n = 198)	90 (n = 203)	NA
Messing et al. (1999)[a] (continuous ± surgery)	38 (n = 51)	83 (n = 41)	NA
Fellow et al. (1992)[a] (continuous ± radiation)	20 (n = 88)	44 (n = 99)	44 (n = 90)
Oliver (2000a)[b] (hormone treatment ± radiation)	NA	50 (n = 11)	38 (n = 15)

[a]Five-year progression free + 5 years free of metastases in randomised trial.
[b]Three years off hormones, non-randomised phase I/II study.

surgical castration. The need for maximum androgen blockade has been increasingly questioned. In these studies surrogate endpoints such as completeness of normalisation of PSA have shown more significant benefit from maximum androgen blockade than overall survival. This could be caused by the stronger selection pressure of total androgen withdrawal producing earlier response at the expense of a more rapid generation of hormone resistance. As a result of these observations and evidence from animal studies suggesting doubling of duration of time to hormone resistance in some (Sato et al. 1996), but not all, models, there has been increasing interest in use of intermittent hormone therapy since 1993. With more than 400 patients studied in phase II trials, results show that the average cycle consists of 9 months on and 9 months off and the average patient remains hormone sensitive for three or more cycles, i.e. 54 months' survival instead of 24–36 months of continuous hormone use. There are now two major randomised trials in progress in patients with M+ diseases, and it should not be long before it is clear whether there is prolonged survival for this strategy.

Where next with intermittent hormone therapy trials for metastatic and localised prostate cancer?

Potential for exploring intermittent hormone therapy cycling time as a surrogate endpoint for screening new agents in patients with metastatic prostate cancer

The published results with intermittent hormone therapy suggest that, in the average patient, cycles of 6–9 months on hormone treatment are followed by the same time off treatment. However, they also demonstrated that between 20 and 40% patients have longer periods of up to 4 years or more off treatment. Although part of this is the result of the association of prolonged hormone treatment with slow recovery of testosterone and the slow rise of PSA, a significant number have normal libido and testosterone levels.

The question that these observations raise is whether it is possible to use the speed of PSA recovery relative to testosterone levels as a surrogate endpoint to investigate new therapies.

Although there is a trend for shorter cycles, the more cycles that the patient goes through (Table 8.8), the more significant observation is the regularity of cycles. This is the most important observation to emerge from the intermittent hormone therapy studies, because the impact of additional therapeutic interventions on duration of cycles offers a considerable potential as an early surrogate endpoint for monitoring new therapeutic interventions. An illustration of this is shown in Table 8.9 where duration of time off hormones has been increased almost threefold after addition of treatment with radiation to cover all areas of known disease. Clearly the numbers are too small for statistical significance, although they do illustrate the potential to screen new treatment by treating 10 patients with intermittent hormone therapy who have had evidence of a short cycle off hormone therapy, and seeing whether it is possible to demonstrate a gain comparable to that achieved in patients with local disease who receive radiotherapy. If this proves successful, it would be easy to proceed to a randomised phase II study with the appropriate number of patients to prove that the observed difference in the pilot study of 10 patients is statistically significant, with patients randomised to the control arm being eligible to receive salvage treatment for the third cycle of intermittent therapy.

Table 8.8 Comparison of first, second and third cycle lengths in intermittent hormone therapy

	Median duration of hormone therapy (months)	Median time off (months)	Mean time off (months)
First cycle (n = 14)	10	11	16
Second cycle (n = 14)	7	7	8.3
3rd cycle (n = 3)	9	6	8.7

Values in parentheses are the ranges.

Table 8.9 Factors influencing duration of second cycle off hormone therapy

		No. of cases	Median duration of first cycle off hormone therapy	Median duration of second cycle off hormone therapy
PSA at start of second cycle	> 25 (25–149)	8	15	11
	≤ 25 (4.4–24)	10	7	7
Radiation consolidation of second cycle	Yes	4	12	20
	No	14	6.2	6
Duration of second cycle hormone therapy (months)	< 9	9	7	7
	≥ 9	9	13	13
Stage at first hormone induction treatment	> T3N0M0	9	9	5
	< T3N0M0	9	11	15

Advanced localised disease – the need for a 2 × 2 study of intermittent monotherapy vs maximum androgen blockade plus immediate vs deferred radiation for M0 prostate cancer unsuitable for surgery

Studies of immediate versus deferred hormone therapy (Anonymous 1997) and with maximum androgen blockade (Crawford *et al.* 1989) provide some support for the view that the benefit from hormone therapy is greatest when used in patients with less advanced prostate cancer in terms of immediate response parameters but not overall survival. Recently, two studies (Small *et al.* 1996; Oliver *et al.* 1997) have suggested that this may also be true in respect of use of intermittent hormone therapy. In our study, 38% of M0 patients have survived relapse free at 36 months after stopping hormone therapy (Table 8.10). However, there is evidence from randomised trials that overall survival is prolonged after using hormones to enhance radiation-induced downstaging (Bolla *et al.* 1997; Pilepich *et al.* 1997) and using hormones

Table 8.10 Impact of M stage and radiation on PSA relapse in patients entered into intermittent hormone therapy studies

Study	No. of cases	Progression free (%) off hormone therapy for			
		1 year	2 years	3 years	4 years
M+ and/or N+ (hormone therapy alone)	19	37	21	7	NA
M0 (HT alone)	16	56	38	38	38
M0 (hormone therapy pre-radiation)	11	90	60	50	20
M0 (hormone therapy, radiation failure)	7	71	36	18	NA

after surgery (Messing *et al.* 1999). As mentioned earlier, in the only trial to compare hormones alone versus radiation plus hormones, albeit grossly underpowered, there was no benefit from immediate addition of radiation (Fellow & Clarke 1992), suggesting that it would be as effective if deferred until relapse.

Possible justification for a large-scale randomised trial to clarify the value of using radiation to consolidate results of primary endocrine therapy in advanced M0 patients receiving intermittent luteinising hormone-releasing hormone (LRHR) analogue therapy, and also to reinvestigate the issues of monotherapy versus maximum androgen blockade, comes from preliminary results of a randomised phase II trial assessing PSA complete response rate and duration of PSA control after immediate versus deferred radiation in patients on intermittent hormone therapy for 6 months. The early results (Oliver *et al.* 2000a) show that initial PSA complete response rate is similar whether or not radiation is given immediately. Although the follow-up is too short to make any observations on the cycle time off hormone therapy, a randomised trial is now under way to investigate this question. A further question that has never been addressed in prostate cancer is whether the combined approach increases the frequency of durable pathological complete response and whether downstaged, but incomplete, responders would benefit from early surgery as in bladder cancer (Blandy *et al.* 1985), before radiation fibrosis makes surgery difficult.

Early localised disease – the need for a feasibility 2 × 2 study of short-term vs long-term intermittent bicalutamide monotherapy plus immediate vs deferred radiation and/or surgery for potentially operable M0 prostate cancer

Recently, there have successful reports from use of continuous bicalutamide (Casodex) monotherapy as an alternative to LHRH analogues in advanced M0 (Iversen *et al.* 1998) and more recently early M0 patients (Abrahamsson 2001) as an adjunct to primary radiation, surgery or surveillance. However, there is evidence in patients on anti-androgen monotherapy that one escape mechanism is a mutant androgen receptor using the anti-androgen as growth factor (Taplin *et al.* 1995). As a result of this, it is possible that, in contrast to the experience from using tamoxifen in breast cancer where 5 years are the norm, there could be greater benefit from use of intermittent short-term rather than continuous bicalutamide monotherapy in M0 patients. This would be so particularly if there were to be an even larger subgroup of patients who survived for more than 2 years off treatments than those seen in advanced disease studies (see Table 8.10). As yet there have been no studies of intermittent anti-androgen monotherapy in early M0 disease because there are worries that the high circulating testosterone levels, which develop from the effects of anti-androgen, could accelerate recurrence. Given that early limited phase I/II experience from use of anti-androgen monotherapy in our intermittent hormone therapy in advanced M0 patients (Oliver *et al.* 2000a) suggests that it may be safe, there could be a case to justify a randomised phase II pilot study to investigate the safety of short-term (9 months) versus long-term (30/60 months) bicalutamide monotherapy combined with immediate versus deferred local therapy, i.e. either radiation or surgery, in older patients with M0 disease in whom the benefits of surgery or radiotherapy is questioned.

If this phase II confirmed the safety of such an intermittent hormone therapy approach, there could then be a case to expand it to a formal phase III 2 × 2 trial of short- versus long-term hormone therapy ± immediate versus deferred local therapy, either radiation or surgery.

What are the potentials of medical therapy for screening and prevention trials?

Despite the European trial of PSA screening now being close to having recruited its target, it will still be at least another 6–8 years before there is any expectation that data will begin to emerge let alone proof that it is beneficial (Gotzsche 2001; Schröder 2001). In addition, despite there being more than 400 patients with good risk prostate cancer randomised between observation and radical prostatectomy in the Swedish study, it will be at least another 1–2 years before actual results will be available.

On this basis it is clear that there is time to explore alternative possible surrogate endpoints in patients with early disease while awaiting the results of these key studies. Three possible options have emerged.

Investigation of a combined STD screen and therapy for bacterial and virological causes for raised PSA and the possibility of reversing false-positive results to improve predictive power of PSA screening

It has been known since a landmark study by Breslow et al. (1977) that the incidence of latent prostate cancer in postmortem examinations of deaths unrelated to prostate cancer increases with age in a similar way in all populations that were examined, whereas deaths from prostate cancer differ markedly with high rates in Africans and low rates in the Far and Middle East (Oishi et al. 1995). Levels are intermediate in Europeans, although higher in European immigrants to North and South America (Morton 1996). Postmortem brain histology studies also demonstrate that the changes of dementia increase at a similar rate to that of latent prostate cancer (Morris 1999).

Recently virological studies have demonstrated possible indirect mechanisms whereby the viruses can kickstart both prostate cancer and degenerative brain disease. In dementia there is some indirect evidence for involvement of herpes simplex virus (HSV). This virus is widespread but usually short-lived. However, in a minority it can become a long-standing persistent infection in nerve cells and is responsible for recurrent cold sores of the lips and genitals. There has been one report showing that, in dementia, persistent herpes virus is found only in the brain if the individual has a particular gene called *ApoE* ε4 (Itzhaki *et al*. 1997). That this may be relevant to prostate cancer has emerged from recent studies which have shown that men with the *ApoE* ε4 gene are more likely to develop prostate cancer (Lehrer 1998). Although there has been some old anti-herpes serology data from the early 1980s suggesting an association between HSV and prostate cancer (Luleci *et al*. 1981), recent data have suggested a more significant association with human papilloma virus (HPV), another sexually transmitted virus (as yet there has been no work done on the effect of combined HPV and HSV infection). These new data, which are almost as significant as the role of HPV in cervix cancer (Nobbenhuis *et al*. 2001), suggest that HPV could play a role 10–20 years before diagnosis in the initiation of prostate cancer (Dillner *et al*. 1998; Griffiths & Mellon 2000). These observations, combined with old data in cattle showing that papilloma viruses often initiate malignant transformation and then are lost from the genome of the tumour (Campo 1985), i.e. they have a 'hit and run' type of role in the malignant process, may explain how HPV could be indirectly involved in prostate cancer development (Oliver *et al*. 1998). Epidemiological evidence demonstrates a significant association between early age of onset of sexual intercourse and multiple episodes of non-specific STDs (Key 1995). Up to 20% of accident victims have evidence of the earliest pre-cancer changes of prostate cancer intraepithelial neoplasia (PIN) by the age of 40 (Sakr *et al*. 1995). A prospective study in 40 year olds in STD and infertility clinics looking for a correlation between blood levels of PSA and the presence of HSV and HPV infection could provide evidence to support the association. It might also be possible to link these studies with screening for candidate prostate cancer-predisposing genes (Rebbeck & Jaffe 1998; Makridakis & Ross 1999) as well as androgen receptor polymorphisms and the *ApoE* ε4 genetic status. Using these and other markers of high risk such as cytogenic changes (see below) could predict more precisely the high-risk patients at a younger age. Early nerve-sparing surgery could be justified in these patients if combined with pelvic floor exercises (Van Kampen *et al*. 2000) to reduce risk of incontinence and impotence.

Investigation of new cytogenetic and molecular screening techniques to improve specificity of PSA screening

Cytogenetics with 24-colour multiple fluorescence *in situ* hybridisation is a new technique developed through the study of primate genetics (Muller *et al*. 2000) and haematological cancer (Cigudosa *et al*. 1998), which is increasingly being applied to adult solid cancer (Melcher *et al*. 2000). Preliminary results from prostate cancer cell lines (Strefford *et al*. 2000) and first passage cultures (Bright *et al*. 1997) are demonstrating that it is a very powerful technique to examine the genetic changes in clonal development of this cancer (Qian *et al*. 1999; Dhanasekran *et al*. 2001). However, the more widespread application of this technology is limited because of the difficulty in getting access to adequate tissue with dividing cells to do routine cytogenetics on primary tissues.

Recently, there have been reports that selective use of bone trephine on bone scan hotspots makes it possible to identify areas of prostate malignancy in more than 90% of biopsies (Hussain *et al*. 1996). Improved monoclonal antibodies to cell membrane-expressed prostate cancer markers for cell sorting (Bander *et al*. 2000) make it possible to separate these cells by cell-sorting techniques. There have also been reports that it is possible to use the E6/E7 construct from HPV 16/17 to develop short-lived cell cultures from prostate cancer biopsies (Choo *et al*. 1999) and new selective media that enhance growth of prostate cells (Fry *et al*. 2000).

If these early reports were to be confirmed, it might be possible to obtain reliable cytogenetic spreads from every patient and use them to score for cytogenetic changes in patients before treatment and after the development of hormone resistance as predictions of clinical behaviour. Given the number of animal models showing a slower progression to hormone resistance when intermittent compared with continuous hormone therapy (Sato *et al*. 1996), it might also be interesting to compare patients in such studies. If it proves possible to develop routine culture techniques for screening prostate biopsies, it might also be possible to apply the techniques to ejaculates. If such a technique could be validated, it would have considerable potential in predicting which PSA-positive patients had an increased risk and might gain most benefit from early surgical intervention.

Use of population-based PSA as a surrogate early endpoint to investigate the impact of a population-based education programme on risk factors for prostate cancers

From evidence that population-based PSA levels give a prediction of risk of death from prostate cancer 10 years before it happens (Parkes *et al*. 1995), sequential population-based PSA sampling would give an early indication of impact of a population-based education programme or therapeutic manoeuvre.

It is clear from the preceding section that there are several important messages for men that could reduce their life-time risk of prostate cancer which need to be learned at the time of puberty, i.e. safe sun, safe sex, good diet and regular exercise.

Setting out to investigate the impact of teenager education about these issues could take 40–50 years before there would be a reduction in deaths from prostate cancer. As one study (Oliver *et al*. 2001) has suggested that population-based PSA blood testing may give an early indication of prostate damage by the age of 25–30, extending these messages into the workplace and to family planning, vasectomy and STD clinics could ensure that the benefit of the message is also reinforced over a wider population. It might then be possible to measure its impact on populations by studying serial PSA levels in blood donors.

Long before the impact of such education campaigns on prostate cancer could be fully evaluated, there would be other interim checkpoints that could highlight the progress being made. The first of these would be a reduction in the incidence of teenage pregnancies, one of the more embarrassing statistics on which the UK leads the rests of Europe. Second, there could be a reduction in STDs – which have recently begun to take off again as the HIV/AIDS threat has seemed to diminish. There could also be a reduction in the early stages of cervix cancer. Third, there might even be a reduction in the occurrence of depression and suicide in young men, because exercise and sunlight have both been shown to reduce risks of these events. Fourth, and by no means least, we might see more UK success in national and international sporting competitions such as the Olympics and the Football World Cup.

Conclusion

Despite stage shift from increasing use of early PSA screening leading to more early stage disease, there is as yet no evidence that surgery or radiation offer any survival advantage over one another or patients treated expectantly. However, at present these modalities remain the standard of care for patients with early disease on rectal examination and with a PSA < 30. In the USA surgery is favoured for the younger patients with PSA < 15 and radiation more frequently used for older patients with a PSA of 15–30, and there is a similar trend in this direction beginning in the UK.

Results after both surgery and radiation are enhanced by hormone therapy when used in combination. However, realisation that there are no trials comparing hormone alone versus the combination is leading to increasing interest in exploring the potential of initially using intermittent hormone therapy in these cases and only using local therapy if there is early recurrence when hormone therapy is stopped.

This review has done the following:

1. Highlighted the long latent period and multiple risk factors involved in the development of prostate cancer and the possibilities of modifying the development by medical intervention long before the onset of life-threatening disease and the value of population-based PSA studies as a surrogate endpoint to assess effect of such intervention.
2. Focused on the potential of intermittent hormone therapy and the outstanding question of the last decade as to whether the laboratory observation from animal studies that it doubles duration of time to hormone resistance actually translates into any discernible clinical benefit.
3. Reviewed the opportunity from use of intermittent hormone therapy in patients with M0 disease and the potential of using off treatment cycle time as a surrogate endpoint to examine new treatment and clarify the value of established treatments such as radiation and surgery.

References

Abrahamsson P (2001). Treatment of locally advanced prostate cancer – A new role for antiandrogen monotherapy? *European Urology* **39**(suppl), 22–28

Albertson PC (2000). Treatment of early stage prostate cancer: expectant management. In Vogelzang NJ, ed., *Comprehensive Textbook of Genito-Urinary Oncology*. 2nd edn. Philadelphia: Lippincott, Williams & Wilkins, pp. 715–721

Anonymous (1997). Immediate versus deferred treatment for advanced prostatic cancer; initial results of the Medical Research Council Trial. The Medical Research Council Prostate Cancer Working Party Investigators Group. *British Journal of Urology* **79**, 235–246

Anonymous (1998). Polychemotherapy for early breast cancer: an overview of the randomised trials. Early Breast Cancer Trialists' Collaborative Group (see comments). *The Lancet* **352**, 930–942

Auvinen A, Vornanen T, Tammela T *et al.* (2001). A randomised trial of choice of treatment in prostate cancer. *British Journal of Urology International* **88**, 708–715

Bander N, Nanus D, Bremer S *et al.* (2000). Phase I clinical trial targeting a monoclonal antibody (mab) to the extracellular domain of prostate specific membrane in patients with hormone-independent prostate cancer. *Proceedings of the American Society of Clinical Oncology* abstract 1872

Bekesi J, Roboz J, Solomno S, Fischvein A, Selikoff I (1983). Persistent immune dysfunction in Michigan dairy farm residents exposed to polybrominated biphenyls. *Immunotox* **1**, 182

Beral V, Inskip H, Fraser P (1985). Mortality of employees of the United Kingdom Atomic Energy Authority 1946–1979. *British Medical Journal* **291**, 440

Blandy JP, Tiptaft RC, Paris AMI, Oliver RTD, Hope-Stone HF (1985). The case for definitive radiotherapy and salvage cystectomy in localised bladder carcinoma. *World Journal of Urology* **3**, 94–97

Bolla M, Gonzalez D, Warde P *et al.* (1997). Improved survival in patients with locally advanced prostate cancer treated with radiotherapy and goserelin. *New England Journal of Medicine* **337**, 295–300

Brabin L (2001). Hormonal markers of susceptibility to sexually transmitted infections: are we taking then seriously? *British Medical Journal* **323**, 394–395

Breslow N, Chan CW, Dhom G *et al.* (1977). Latent carcinoma of prostate at autopsy in seven areas. *International Journal of Cancer* **20**, 680–688

Bright R, Vocke C, Emmert-Buck M *et al.* (1997). Generation and genetic characterization of immortal human prostate epithelial cell lines derived from primary cancer specimens. *Cancer Research* **57**, 995–1002

Campo M, Moor M, Satirana M *et al.* (1985). Bovine papilloma virus 4 for maintenance of alimentary cancers in cattle. *EMBO J* **4**, 1819–1825

Chodak G & Palmer JS (1996). Defining the role of surveillance in the management of localised prostate cancer. *Urologic Clinics of North America* **23**, 551–556s

Choo C, Ling M, Chan K *et al.* (1999). Immortalization of human prostate epithelial cells by HPV 16 E6/E7 open reading frames. *Prostate* **40**, 150–158

Cigudosa J, Road P, Calasanz M *et al.* (1998). Characterization of nonrandom chromosomal gains and losses in multiple myeloma by comparative genomic hybridization. *Blood* **91**, 3007–3010

Clark LC, Combs GF Jr, Turnbull BW *et al.* (1996). Effects of selenium supplementation for cancer prevention in patients with carcinoma of the skin. A randomized controlled trial. Nutritional Prevention of Cancer Study Group. *Journal of the American Medical Association* **276**, 1957–1963

Corder EH, FRiedman GD, Vogelman J, Orenteich N (1993). Risk of prostate cancer and serum 1,25-D vitamin D metabolite level. *Cancer Epidemiology Biomarkers and Prevention* **2**, 467–473

Crabtree JE, Wyatt JI, Trejdosiewicz LK *et al.* (1994). Interleukin-8 expression in *Helicobacter pylori* infected, normal, and neoplastic gastroduodenal mucosa. *Journal of Clinical Pathology* **47**, 61–6

Crawford E, Eisenberger M, McLead D *et al.* (1989). A controlled trial of leuprolide with and without flutamide in prostatic carcinoma. *New England Journal of Medicine* **321**, 419–424

Danesh J, Newton R, Beral V (1997). A human germ project. *Nature* **389**, 21–24

Davies PD (1995). Tuberculosis and migration. The Mitchell Lecture 1994. *Journal of the Royal College of Physicians of London* **29**(2), 113–118

Dhanasekran SM, Rubin M, Chinnaiyan AM *et al.* (2001). Delineation of prognostic biomarkers in prostate cancer. *Nature* **412**, 822–826

Dillner J, Knekt P, Boman J *et al.* (1998). Sero-epidemiological association between human papillomavirus infection and risk of prostate cancer. *International Journal of Cancer* **75**, 564–567

Fellow G & Clark P (1992). Treatment of advanced localised prostate cancer by orchidectomy, radiotherapy or combination therapy. *British Journal of Urology* **70**, 304–309

Fleming LE, Bean JA, Rudolph M, Hamilton K (1999). Mortality in licenced pesticide applicatory in Florida. *Occupational and Environmental Medicine* **56**, 14–21

Fossa S, Eri L, Skovlund E *et al.* (2001). No randomised trial of prostate cancer screening in Norway. *Journal of Oncology* **2**, 741–745

Forman D (1996). *Helicobacter pylori* and gastric cancer. *Scandinavian Journal of Gastoenterology* **31**, 48–51

Fry P, Hudson D, O'Hare M, Masters J (2000). Comparison of marker protein expression in benign hyperplasia in vivo and in vitro. *British Journal of Urology International* **85**, 504–513

Gajalakshmi C & Shanta V (1993). Association between cervical and penile cancers in Madras, India. *Acta Oncologica* **32**, 617–620

Gerbase AC, Rowley JT, Mertens TE (1998). Global epidemiology of sexually transmitted diseases. *The Lancet* **351**(suppl 3), 2–4

Giovannucci E, Ascherio A, Rimm EB, Stampfer MJ, Colditz GA, Willett WC (1995). Intake of carotenoids and retinol in relation to risk of prostate cancer. *Journal of the National Cancer Institute* **87**, 1767–1776

Gleave M, La Bianca S, Goldenberg SL (2000). Neoadjuvant hormonal therapy prior to radical prostatectomy: promises and pitfalls. *Prostate Cancer and Prostatic Diseases* **7**, 136–144

Gotzsche PC (2001). Debate on screening for breast cancer is not over. *British Medical Journal* **323**, 693

Granfors T, Modig H, Danbar J, Tomice R (1998). Orchidectomy and radiotherapy versus radiotherapy for prostate cancer. *Journal of Urology* **159**, 2030–2034

Griffiths T & Mellon J (2000). Human papillomavirus and urological tumours: II. Role in bladder, prostate, renal and testicular cancer. *British Journal of Urology International* **85**, 211–217

Hanchette C & Schwartz (1992). Inverse correlation between UV radiation exposure in USA and Prostate cancer mortality. *Cancer* **70**, 2861–2869)

Hayes RB, Ziegler RG, Gridley G *et al*. (1999). Dietary factors and risks for prostate cancer among blacks and whites in the United States. *Cancer Epidemiology Biomarkers and Prevention* **8**(1), 25–34

Heshmat M, Kovi J, Herson J, Jones G, Jackson M (1975). Epidemiologic association between gonorrhea and prostatic carcinoma. *Urology* **6**, 457–460

Hussain M, Kukuruga M, Biggar S, Sakr W, Cummings G, Ensley J (1996). Prostate cancer: flow cytometric methods for detection of bone marrow micrometastases. *Cytometry* **26**, 40–46

Itzhaki R, Lin W, Shang D, Wilcock G, Faragher B, Jamieson G (1997). Herpes simplex virus type 1 in brain and risk of Alzheimer's disease (see comments). *The Lancet* **349**, 241–244

Iversen P, Madsen PO, Corle DK (1995). Radical prostatectomy versus expectant treatment for early carcinoma of the prostate. Twenty-three year follow-up of a prospective randomized study. *Scandinavian Journal of Urology and Nephrology* suppl 172, 65–72

Iversen P, Tyrrell CJ, Kaisary A *et al*. (1998). Casodex (bicalutamide) 150-mg monotherapy compared with castration in patients with previously untreated non-metastatic prostate cancer: Results from two multi-centre randomised trials at a median follow-up of 4 years. *Urology* **51**, 389–396

Key T (1995). Risk factors for prostate cancer. *Cancer Surveys* **23**, 63–77

Kirk D (1996). Hormone therapy in advanced prostate cancer – report of the Medical Research Council 'immediate' verses 'deferred' treatment study. *British Journal of Urology* **77**(suppl) (abstr 204)

Kuban DA, Schellhammer, Paul F, El-Mahdi, Anas M (2000). External-beam radiation therapy for stage t1 and t2 prostate cancer. In Vogetzany NJ, ed., *Comprehensive Textbook of Genito-Urinary Oncology*, 2nd edn. Philadelphia: Lippincott, Williams & Wilkins, pp 739–753

Lehrer S (1998). Possible relationship of the apoliprotein E (apo E) Ee4 allele to prostate cancer. *British Journal of Cancer* **78**, 1398

Luleci G, Sakizli M, Gunalp A, Erkan I, Remzi D (1981). Herpes simplex type 2 neutralization antibodies in patients with cancers of urinary bladder, prostate and cervix. *Journal of Surgical Oncology* **16**, 327–331

Luscombe J, Fryer AA, French ME *et al*. (2001). Exposure to ultraviolet radiation: association with susceptibility and age at presentation with prostate cancer. *The Lancet* **358**, 641–642

Makridakis N & Ross RK (1999). Association of mis-sense substitution in SRD5A2 gene with prostate cancer in African-American and Hispanic men in Los Angeles, USA. *The Lancet* **354**, 975–978

Melcher R, Steinlein C, Feichtinger W *et al*. (2000). Spectral karyotyping of the human colon cancer cell lines SW480 and SW620. *Cytogenetics and Cell Genetics* **88**, 145–152

Messing E, Manola J, Sarosdy M, Wilding G, Crawford E, Trump D (1999). Immediate hormonal therapy compared with observation after radical prostatectomy and pelvic lymphadenectomy in men with node-positive prostate cancer. *New England Journal of Medicine* **341**, 1215–1216

Mettlin C, Murphy GP, Rosenthal DS, Menck HR (1998). The National Cancer Data Base report on prostate carcinoma after the peak in incidence rates in the US. *Cancer* **83**, 1679–1684

Meyer F, Bairati I, Shadmani R, Fradet Y, Moore L (1999). Dietary fat and prostate cancer survival. *Cancer Causes and Control* **10**, 245–251

Morris J (1999). Is Alzheimer's disease inevitable with age? Lessons with clinicopathologic studies of health aging and very mild Alzheimer's disease. *Journal of Clinical Investigation* **104**, 1171

Morton R (1996). Prostate cancer in ethnic groups. In Vogelzang N, Scardino P, Shipley W, Coffey D (eds) *Comprehensive Textbook of Genitourinary Oncology.* Philadelphia: Williams & Wilkins, pp. 573–578

Muller S, O'Brien P, Ferguson-Smith M, Wienberg J (2000). Cross-species colour segmenting: a novel tool in human karyotype analysis. *Cytometry* **33**, 445–452

Nakata S, Imai K, Yamanaka H (1993). Study of risk factors for prostatic cancer (Japanese). *Hinyokika Kiyo* **39**, 1017–1024

Nobbenhuis M, Helmerhorst T, van der Brule A *et al.* (2001). Cytological regression of high risk HPV. *The Lancet* **358**, 1782–1783

O'Byrne K, Dalgleish A, Browning M, Steward W, Harris A (2000). The relationship between angiogenesis and the immune response in carcinogenesis and the progression of malignant disease. *European Journal of Cancer* **36**, 151–169

Oishi K, Yoshida O, Schroeder F (1995). The geography of prostate cancer and its treatment in Japan. *Cancer Surveys* **23**, 267–280

Oliver JC, Oliver RTD, Ballard RC (2001). Influence of circumcision and sexual behaviour on PSA levels in patients attending a STD clinic. *Prostate Cancer and Prostate Diseases* **4**, 228–231

Oliver R (1995). Prostate cancer: a physician's perspective. *Cancer Surveys* **23**, 309–310

Oliver R (2000). Intermittent hormone therapy: its potential in early prostate cancer and intra-epithelial neoplasia. In Belldegrun A, Kirby R, Newling D (eds) *New Perspectives in Prostate Cancer.* Oxford: Isis Medical Media Ltd, pp. 223–227

Oliver R, Belldegrun A, Wrigley P (1995). Preventing prostate cancer: Screening verses chemotherapy – pros and cons based on new views of its biology, early events and clinical behaviour – introduction. *Cancer Surveys* **23**, 1–3

Oliver R, Grant-Williams G, Paris A, Blandy J (1997). Intermittent androgen deprivation after PSA complete as a strategy to reduce induction of hormone resistant prostate cancer. *Urology* **49**, 79–82

Oliver RTD, Breuer J, Nouri AME, Campo S (1998). Malignancy associated papillomaviruses and morphology of human bladder cancer. *Cancer Surveys* **27**, 29–47

Oliver R, Farrugia D, Ansell W, Chinegwundoh F (2000a). Potential of intermittent hormone therapy for M+ and M0 prostate cancer patients. *Prostate Cancer and Prostatic Diseases* **3**, 286–289

Oliver S, Gunnel D, Donovan J (2000b). Comparison of trends in prostate cancer mortality in England and Wales and the USA. *The Lancet* **355**, 1788–1789

Oliveria SA, Kohl HW, Trichopoulous D, Blair SN (1996). The association between cardiorespiratory fitness and prostate cancer. *Medical Science and Sports Exercise* **28**, 97–104

Parkes C, Wald N, Murphy P *et al.* (1995). Prospective observational study to asses value of prostate cancer in England and Wales. *British Journal of Urology* **79**, 97–104

Petrikowski CG, Pharoah MJ, Lee L, Grace MG (1995). Radiographic differentiation of osteogenic sarcoma, osteomyelitis, and fibrous dysplasia of the jaws. *Oral Surgery, Oral Medicine, Oral Pathology and Oral Radiology and Endodontics* **80**, 744–750

Pilepich M, Caplan R, Byhardt R *et al.* (1997). Androgen deprivation with radiation-therapy compared with radiation-therapy alone for locally advanced prostatic-carcinoma – a randomised comparative trial of the radiation-therapy oncology group. *Journal of Clinical Oncology* **5**, 1013–1021

Qian J, Jenkins RB, Bostwick DG (1999). Genetic and chromosomal alterations in prostatic intraepithelial neoplasia and carcinoma detected by fluorescence in situ hybridization. *European Urology* **35**, 479–483

Rebbeck T & Jaffe JM (1998). Modification of clinical presentation of prostate tumours by a novel genetic variant in CYP3A4. *Journal of the National Cancer Institute* **90**, 1225–1229

Roberts R, Lieber M, Rhodes T, Girman C, Bostwick D, Jacobsen S (1998). Prevalence of a physician assigned diagnosis of prostatitis: the Olmstead County Study of Urinary Symptoms and Health Status Among Men. *Urology* **51**, 578–584

Ross R, Shimizi H, Paganini-Hill A, Honda G, Henderson B (1987). Case-control studies of prostate cancer in blacks and whites in southern California. *Journal of the National Cancer Institute* **78**, 869–874

Ross R, Bernstein L, Lobo R (1992a). 5-alpha-reductase activity and risk of prostate cancer among Japanese and US white and black males. *The Lancet* **339**, 887–889

Ross RK, Yuan JM, Yu MC *et al.* (1992b). Urinary aflatoxin and hepatocellular carcinoma. *The Lancet* **339**, 943–946

Rotkin I (1967). Adolescent coitus and cervical cancer associations of related events with increased risk. *Cancer Research* **27**, 603–617

Sakr WA, Grignon DJ, Hass G *et al.* (1995). Epidemiology of high grade intraepithelial neoplasia. *Pathology, Research and Practice* **191**, 838–841

Sato N, Gleave ME, Bruchovsky N (1996). Intermittent androgen suppression delays progression to androgen-independent regulation of prostate-specific antigen gene in the LNCap prostate tumour model. *Journal of Steroid Biochemistry and Molecular Biology* **58**, 139–146

Schmitz-Drager BJEM, Beiche B, Ebert T (2001). Nutrition and prostate cancer. *Urologia Internationalis* **67**(1), 1–11

Schroder FH (2001). Diagnosis, characterisation and potential clinical relevance of prostate cancer detected at low PSA ranges. *European Urology* **39**(4), 49–53

Semba R, Muhilal, Ward B *et al.* (1993). Abnormal T cell subset proportions in Vitamin A deficient children. *The Lancet* **341**, 5–8

Small E, Grossfeld G, Carroll P (1996). Intermittent androgen deprivation for clinically localised prostate cancer. *Proceedings of the American Society of Clinical Oncology* **16**, 343a (abstract 1225)

Strefford J, Young B, Oliver R (2000). The use of multi-colour fluorescence technologies in the characterisation of prostate carcinoma cell line: A comparison of multi-plex FISH and spectral karyotyping data. *Cancer Genetics and Cytogenetics* **124**, 112–121

Strum S, McDermed JE, Scholz M, Johnson H, Tisman G (1997). Anaemia associated with androgen deprivation in patients with prostate cancer receiving combined hormone blockade. *British Journal of Urology* **79**, 933–941

Taplin M, Bubley G, Shuster T *et al.* (1995). Mutation of the androgen receptor gene in metastatic androgen-independent prostate cancer. *New England Journal of Medicine* **332**, 1393–1398

Van Kampen M, De Weerdt W, Van Poppel H, De Ridder D, Feys H, Baert L (2000). Effect of pelvic-floor re-education on duration and degree of incontinence after radical prostatectomy: a randomised controlled trial. *The Lancet* **355**, 98–102

Warming B (1986). Condoms in Japan (letter). *Nature* **332**, 10

Wei J, Gross M, Jaffe C *et al.* (1999). Androgen deprivation therapy for prostate cancer results in significant loss of bone density. *Urology* **54**, 607–611

Wirth M, See WA, McLeod DG, Iversen P (2001). The bicalutamide early prostate cancer program. *Urology and Oncology* **6**, 43–47

Yeole BB & Jussawalla DJ (1997). Descriptive epidemiology of the cancers of male genital organs in greater Bombay. *Indian Journal of Cancer* **34**(1), 30–39

Zietman A, Prince E, Nakfoor B, Dark J (1997). Androgen deprivation and radiation therapy: sequencing studies using serotinergic tumour system. *International Journal of Radiation Oncology, Biology, Physics* **38**, 1067–1070

Chapter 9

The medical management of advanced prostatic cancer

Andreas Polychronis and R Tim D Oliver

In the Western World, prostate cancer is the cause of more than 1% of all deaths in men. It is the most common cancer diagnosed in men and, after lung cancer, is the second most common cause of cancer death in men (Parker *et al*. 1996). Its incidence is increasing by 2–3% per year. There are two main reasons for this increase. The first is increased life expectancy and the second is that prostate-specific antigen (PSA) testing has enabled earlier, and more accurate, diagnosis of the disease. The general prognosis for prostate cancer remains poor, with 70% survival at 10 years compared with the general population. About half of all cases are diagnosed at a locally advanced stage and about 30% have bone metastases at the time of diagnosis (Petrovich *et al*. 1997).

In the UK, 21,400 new cases were diagnosed in 1996 and 9,460 deaths were reported in 1998. The latter figure represents 19% of all UK cancer deaths (Office for National Statistics 1999). In the USA, 317,000 new cases were diagnosed in 1997 and 41,000 deaths recorded (Parker *et al*. 1996). There is an even larger number of patients annually who, during the course of their disease, develop metastases after a course of definitive treatment for organ-confined disease such as radical prostatectomy or pelvic irradiation. However, the 33rd annual compilation of cancer statistics (1999) showed that the incidence of prostate cancer had decreased significantly with a reduction in death rate of 11% since 1991 (Landis *et al*. 1999). These statistics also reported an increase of 20% in 10-year survival between 1988 and 1995.

Prognostic factors in patients with advanced disease

The rates of prostate cancer progression and survival time vary tremendously from patient to patient. The median overall survival for all patients treated with hormone therapies is about 30 months (Galbraith & Duchesne 1997). Patients with low-volume disease and good performance status will generally live longer than those with extensive disease and poor performance status (Crawford *et al*. 1989; Eisenberger *et al*. 1994). Other factors indicating a poor prognosis include the presence of non-axial bone disease, visceral disease, low serum levels of testosterone, elevated serum alkaline phosphatase level, anaemia and symptoms such as pain and weight loss (Crawford *et al*. 1989; Mulders *et al*. 1990; Chodak *et al*. 1991; Eisenberger *et al*. 1994; Robson & Dawson 1996). In addition, patients treated with hormone therapy whose serum

PSA levels do not return to normal within 6 months have a worse prognosis (Matzkin *et al.* 1992; Miller *et al.* 1992; Eisenberger *et al.* 1994). Interestingly, the pre-treatment serum PSA level does not appear to have prognostic significance in patients with metastatic disease and, likewise, the rate of elevation of serum PSA level may not correlate with outcome (Robson & Dawson 1996; Scher *et al.* 1996).

Hormone-sensitive prostate cancer

Approximately three-quarters of metastatic prostate cancers are hormone sensitive. The average time for response to androgen deprivation is about 18 months; survival after second-line treatment varies from 6 to 10 months (Small & Vogelzang 1997).

Early versus late therapy

For symptomatic patients or those with progressive disease, hormonal manipulation is essential. However, for asymptomatic patients this may not necessarily be the case. The unwanted side effects (particularly of a sexual nature) and considerable cost of hormonal therapy are important considerations in initiating such treatments. Also, hormonal treatment continues to remain effective in asymptomatic patients. However, delaying treatment by just 9 months significantly increases the risk of spinal cord compression. Crawford *et al.* (1997a, 1997b) have shown that 45% of prostate cancer patients have regarded quality of life as more important against 29% who stated a preference for prolonged survival. The MRC trial comparing early versus delayed treatment demonstrated, for the first time, the benefits of early treatment in terms of metastatic progression, complications and cancer-related deaths (Medical Research Council Prostate Cancer Working Party Investigators Group 1997).

Androgen deprivation

For about 50 years, androgen deprivation therapy has been the most important and most effective systemic therapy for patients with advanced prostate cancer (Huggins & Hodges 1972). This therapy began to be the recommended treatment for advanced carcinoma of the prostate in 1941, when Huggins and Hodges (1941) demonstrated that prostate cancer cells depend on androgenic stimuli, and that castration or oestrogen treatment causes tumour regression. This can be achieved by castration using oestrogens such as diethylstilbestrol (DES) or more recently using anti-androgens and luteinising hormone-releasing hormone (LHRH) agonists. This treatment reduces the plasma level of testosterone by 95%. Androgen deprivation is, however, associated with a number of possible side effects, namely decreased libido, impotence, hot flushes, osteoporosis, fatigue, hair loss, anaemia, psychological morbidity and, occasionally, breast tenderness.

Castration

For a long period of time, bilateral orchidectomy was the gold standard therapy for effective ablation of testicular androgens. This relatively simple surgical procedure, within 3 hours of completion, typically results in a 95% reduction of the circulating testosterone down to a level of 10–50 ng/100 ml (Daneshgari & Crawford 1993). Orchidectomy is a very well-tolerated procedure, is associated with a low cost and avoids the need to rely on patients' compliance in adhering to prescribed medical therapy. Medical (chemical) castration by LHRH agonists, such as goserelin, leuprorelin, buserelin and triptorelin, is nowadays a more common approach. These drugs have long half-lives and are as effective in their anti-androgen effect as oestrogens or orchidectomy (Chodak 1989). These treatments may sometimes induce a paradoxical effect described as 'tumour flare'. This effect is more frequent in cases involving bone lesions and is the result of initial, temporary increases in levels of LH and testosterone. These may lead to bone pains that last for about a week, or in the worst scenario to spinal cord compression if vertebral metastases are present. This phenomenon explains the need for an anti-androgen that must be taken for 2 weeks before and after medical castration in order to avoid 'tumour flare'.

Oestrogens

Treatment with DES 3 mg/day is also a very efficient therapy in suppressing plasma testosterone levels to a range similar to that seen after castration. They influence the pituitary axis (reduce LH production), adrenal secretion and 5α-reductase activity. The most serious side effects of DES are the cardiovascular complications, which are clearly dose dependent as was demonstrated in a randomised study conducted by the Veterans Administration Cooperative Urological Research Group (1967), which started in 1967. These include pulmonary embolism (4% of patients), deep vein thrombosis (4%), myocardial infarction (3%), cerebrovascular accidents (2%) and peripheral oedema (15–20%) (Daneshgari & Crawford 1993). These complications occurred at a dose of DES of 5 mg/day. At this dose, the benefits obtained by DES appear to be outweighed by side effects (Byar & Corle 1988). These results have led to the use of lower doses of DES, even as low as 1 mg/day (Daneshgari & Crawford 1993). These doses have resulted in therapeutic benefits, although it appears that the threshold dose of 3 mg/day is necessary to obtain maximum androgen blockade. Estramustine phosphate, which is another oestrogen, has the advantage both of having hormonal steroidal properties and of functioning as a nitrogen mustard alkylating agent. It interacts with tubulin, resulting in depolymerisation of microtubules. In addition, it demonstrates a cytotoxic action by binding to the nuclear matrix (Tew & Stearns 1987; Dahllof *et al.* 1993).

Anti-androgens

The mode of action of this group of agents is to block the effect of androgens at the target cell level, i.e. the androgen receptors of the prostate cells. Included in this group are non-steroidal anti-androgens, which are true anti-androgens, and steroidal anti-androgens, which also exhibit progesterone-like activity. Steroid anti-androgens inhibit the release of pituitary LH, decreasing plasma levels of testosterone, and partially inhibit 5α-reductase. These include cyproterone acetate and megestrol acetate, which also block the prostate cell androgen receptors.

The non-steroidal anti-androgens are pure anti-androgens. They are competitive inhibitors of dihydrotestosterone (a very active metabolite of testosterone) on the androgen receptors. They include flutamide, nilutamide and bicalutamide (Blackledge *et al.* 1996). They do not reduce, and may even increase, the plasma levels of testosterone, and hence may result in preserved libido.

Maximum androgen blockade

Prostatic cells are androgen dependent and this is particularly so for a very active metabolite of testosterone, dihydrotestosterone (DHT). There are two pathways responsible for the conversion of testosterone to DHT. One route relies on the action of the enzyme 5α-reductase which converts testosterone to DHT. The other route involves production of dihydroepiandosterone by the adrenal glands. This is converted to testosterone and then DHT in the prostate.

The combination of an LHRH agonist with an anti-androgen results in maximum androgen blockade (MAB) at both testicular and adrenal levels. The concept of the combination of an anti-androgen with an LHRH agonist was introduced in 1982 by Labrie *et al.* (1982, 1985). This group demonstrated marked improvement in response and survival for the combination of castration (medical or surgical) and flutamide, in patients with advanced carcinoma of the prostate; 87 patients were recruited on this study and a positive objective response was reported for all of them. Disease progression after the initial response was seen in eight (9%) patients. The 2-year probability of survival and continuous response were 91% and 81%, respectively. In the group of seven patients who had orchidectomy alone, four (57%) died of carcinoma of the prostate during the observation period ($p < 0.05$).

In support of these findings, the first randomised National Cancer Institute study that took place in 1989 was reported (Crawford *et al.* 1989). In this study, 603 stage II patients were randomised between castration with leuprorelin and flutamide and receiving a placebo. The results demonstrated an improvement in the rate of progression (13.6 vs 16.5 months), and a marked improvement in overall survival (28.3 vs 35.6 months) in the MAB arm ($p = 0.035$). These results were later confirmed by a phase III study of the European Organization for Research and Treatment of Cancer (EORTC) (Denis *et al.* 1993). This reported a similar improvement in survival time of 7.3 months ($p = 0.02$), in favour of a combination of flutamide with LHRH agonist compared with orchidectomy alone.

However, a second study of 1,387 stage II patients treated with orchidectomy and flutamide versus placebo, reported in 1995, again by Crawford and colleagues, failed to show such a clear difference in the reduction of PSA or in the progression-free survival (33 vs 30 months). A meta-analysis of 25 trials comparing castration to MAB, published in the same year, failed to show significant difference between the two groups (5-year survival rate: 22.8% vs 26.2%; $p = 0.0512$) (Prostate Cancer Trialists' Collaborative Group 1995).

Further trials were conducted to compare the different ways of achieving MAB. The long-term effects of using oestrogens and LHRH agonists compared with bilateral orchidectomy do not seem to be the same (Crawford et al. 1998). The trials that show a significant benefit with MAB in terms of survival implemented medical castration as opposed to orchidectomy. LHRH agonists, as well as oestrogens, have a direct cytotoxic effect on prostate cancer cells (Limonta et al. 1992). Furthermore, the association of LHRH agonists with anti-androgens appears to be synergistic. Indeed, investigations of receptors to LHRH on immortal lines of prostate cancer cells have shown that the combination of LHRH agonists with anti-androgens has greater inhibition powers than each one of them alone acting on androgen-sensitive or -resistant lines (Crawford et al. 1998).

A meta-analysis of published randomised controlled trials using non-steroidal anti-androgens included nine studies and established the benefits of MAB in terms of objective response, progression-free survival and overall survival (Caubet et al. 1997). They concluded that there are no statistically significant differences in all these parameters, but in the context of MAB the use of LHRH agonists with non-steroidal anti-androgens appears to be the better option.

Flutamide is the reference anti-androgen. A recent randomised trial of 813 patients compared flutamide with bicalutamide in combination therapy. The outcome favoured bicalutamide with regard to tolerance (lower incidence of diarrhoea), but showed identical progression-free and overall survival (Schellhammer et al. 1997). Also, bicalutamide, as a single agent (> 150 mg/day), is active after the failure of flutamide, although the contrary has not been proven (Schellhammer et al. 1997). The non-steroidal anti-androgen cyproterone acetate has never shown any benefits in survival when associated with medical castration (Thorpe et al. 1996), although when compared with flutamide in MAB schedules it was associated with a longer median survival (Schellhammer et al. 1997).

Intermittent therapy

The rationale behind intermittent therapy is to allow the tumour to repopulate with androgen-sensitive cells after androgen deprivation therapy is stopped. Some investigators have suggested that hormone therapy be stopped when the PSA level normalises and that treatment should be re-started once PSA starts to rise again (Akakura et al. 1993). These investigators consider that apoptosis is hormone dependent and the tumour can grow even in the absence of testosterone. Androgens are thought to suppress certain genes that permit continuous cell growth. With anti-androgen therapy, these genes are activated, allowing the tumour to grow continuously, stimulated by other factors. Withdrawing anti-androgens suppresses these genes again, thus rendering the tumour androgen dependent once more. This approach appears to improve the patients' quality of life along with associated obvious economic benefits (Akakura *et al.* 1993).

Anti-androgen withdrawal

Withdrawal of anti-androgen from combination therapy in patients with progressive disease can lead to a major decrease in PSA levels. Three studies reported by Small and Vogelzang (1997), involving 139 patients on flutamide with progressive disease, have demonstrated that withdrawal of flutamide resulted in a PSA reduction in 21% of cases with a median response of 3.5–5 months. Patients who demonstrated a prolonged response to flutamide are more likely to respond to its withdrawal (Scher & Kelly 1993). When flutamide was combined with another hormonal agent, the response appeared more marked when this latter treatment was given at the start of flutamide rather than later. Therefore, it seems logical to suggest the withdrawal of flutamide when it has been used alone or in combination therapy earlier on, and especially when it has been used for a long time (> 18 months). It has been postulated that this phenomenon is secondary to a possible gene amplification of androgen receptors (Visakorpi *et al.* 1995) or mutations of the androgen receptor genes (Taplin *et al.* 1995).

Androgen deprivation

Surgical or medical adrenalectomy with aminoglutethimide and hydrocortisone shows a less than 10% objective response. Similar response figures are obtained with ketoconazole, which needs high doses that are poorly tolerated (Daneshgari & Crawford 1993). Suramin, a polysulphonated naphthylurea initially used in the treatment of onchocerciasis, decreases testosterone levels and suppresses the production of adrenal steroids. Suramin gives objective response rates between 35% and 54%, but exhibits significant nephro- and neurotoxicity (Eisenberg *et al.* 1995). Its duration of response is usually short – about 5 months (Matzkin & Soloway 1992).

Oestrogens

Increasing dosage of oestrogens in patients who become refractory to this therapy may result in further disease regression. Higher oestrogen doses may have a direct cytotoxic effect on the prostate cancer cells. Fosfestrol is less cardiotoxic than DES and can be given intravenously, resulting in a more rapid uptake (Kristiansen *et al.* 1988). It is a prodrug that is metabolised to DES within the prostate cancer cells and hence exhibits very low plasma levels. This results in low cardiotoxicity. The objective response rates reported are of the order of 40% and the median survival of the responders is 19.6 months versus 4.2 months for the non-responders (Grise *et al.* 1998).

Anti-aromatases

The enzyme aromatase converts cholesterol to pregnenolone. Inhibition of this enzyme by aminoglutethimide stops the synthesis of adrenal steroids as does ketoconazole at high doses (Small & Vogelzang 1997). Other aromatase inhibitors, such as letrozole and anastrozole, are currently under investigation. Similarly, low doses of steroids may produce some response by inhibiting the activity of the adrenal glands (Berry *et al.* 1979).

Hormone-refractory prostate cancer

Chemotherapy is of limited value in the management of patients with advanced carcinoma of the prostate, who become refractory to hormonal therapies (Catalona 1994). Indeed, no randomised study has been able to demonstrate a survival advantage with chemotherapy (Eisenberger & Abrams 1988; Dawson 1993; Scher 1998). Several trials have been conducted over the last 20 years, none of which recruited more than 100 patients. The quality-of-life evaluation criteria have also been somewhat modified (Scher 1998), making evaluation of trial results difficult.

A number of phase III trials have evaluated the role of several chemotherapeutic agents (vinblastine, cyclophosphamide, mitoxantrone/mitozantrone, doxorubicin), including newer ones (taxanes, platinum, oral fluoropyrimidines) administered sequentially, in combination or in simultaneous combination with hormonal therapy (estramustine) (Table 9.1). There have been several American studies suggesting that combination chemotherapy, particularly with estramustine, produces superior response rates compared with chemotherapy alone (Ellerhorst *et al.* 1997). However, these studies have not taken into consideration response to conventional oestrogen, such as stilboestrol, in patients who have failed LHRH analogues. In addition, when stilboestrol is combined with steroids, there is a suggestion that the response rate may be even higher (Farrugia *et al.* 2000). As many of the recent chemotherapy/estramustine combinations are studying taxanes, high-dose steroids are given weekly, and there is some suggestion that dexamethasone as a single agent is better than prednisolone or hydrocortisone (Morioka *et al.* 2002) (Table 9.1).

Evaluation of response to these agents should, however, be reported with caution (Scher *et al.* 1995). Previous treatments should be taken into account, e.g. bicalutamide produces superior response rates when administered after flutamide than after surgical castration. Steroid therapy, which is widely used as antiemetic treatment with chemotherapy, produces a 20–40% response rate alone (Tannock *et al.* 1989). The interval between the end of hormone therapy and the start of chemotherapy should be considered to account for the withdrawal effect. The response to

Table 9.1 Hormone-refractory prostate cancer: second-line treatment with medical therapy

Agents	PSA response > 50%	Objective response
Cyclophosphamide	–	20
Doxorubicin (20 mg/m^2 per week)	39	5–33
Doxorubicin + cyclophosphamide	–	46
Vinblastine	3	5
Paclitaxel	–	5
Docetaxel	41–46	24
Mitoxantrone/mitozantrone	16	–
Mitoxantrone/mitozantrone + prednisolone	20	–
Cyclophosphamide + prednisolone + diethylstilbestrol (DES)	39	–
Doxorubicin + ketoconazole	55	58
Estramustine alone	21	–
Estramustine + vinblastine (VLB)	25–54	–
Estramustine + VLB/doxorubicin + ketoconazole	67	75
Estramustine + etoposide	58	46
Estramustine + paclitaxel	53	28
Estramustine + paclitaxel + etoposide	52	–
Estramustine + docetaxel	60–80	31
Hydrocortisone	19	–
Prednisolone	27	–
Stilboestrol alone	57	–
Dexamethasone alone	62	–
Stilboestrol + hydrocortisone	78	–

withdrawal usually occurs within 4–8 weeks (Small & Vogelzang 1997). The plasma levels of testosterone should also be shown to be equivalent to surgical castration, before commencing chemotherapy (Scher 1998).

A randomised study of 192 patients (Hudes *et al.* 1997) compared vinblastine alone versus vinblastine and estramustine. The response rates were 6% and 18% with a progression-free survival (PFS) of 1.9 and 3.7 months ($p = 0.001$) and an overall survival (OS) of 9.2 and 11.9 months ($p = 0.18$), respectively. This represents a 25% increase in OS, although this is not statistically significant.

Even if there is no gain in OS with chemotherapy, there are benefits in terms of improvement of quality of life. In a randomised study of 161 patients, Tannock *et al.* (1996) compared prednisolone (10 mg/day) with a prednisolone and mitoxantrone combination (12 mg/m^2 every 21 days) as second-line therapy in patients with hormone-refractory carcinoma of the prostate. The objective response rate reported was 29% for the combination versus 12%, median response of 43 weeks versus 18 weeks, and an overall benefit of 38% for the combination versus 21% for the patients treated with prednisolone alone. All these values reached statistical significance. Among those patients who failed with prednisolone alone, the addition of mitoxantrone produced a 22% response rate with a median of 18 weeks. Overall survivals were identical, with a median of 11 months, but 50 of 80 patients treated with prednisolone alone relapsed and then received mitoxantrone in combination with prednisolone. There was an improvement in pain control and overall quality of life. The latter was improved significantly in the combination-therapy group, as assessed by two different quality-of-life instruments (EORTC QLQ-30 and QOLM-P14) (Osoba et al. 1999). The reported toxicities were also acceptable (two cardiac failures among 130 patients treated with mitoxantrone).

Another different but interesting approach was demonstrated by Ellerhorst et al. (1997), in a phase II trial of alternating weekly chemohormone therapy (one week with ketoconazole and doxorubicin and the other with estramustine and vinblastine) combined with daily hydrocortisone. There was a 75% objective response rate in patients with measured disease, a reduction in plasma PSA by more than 50% in 67% of patients and by more than 80% in 52% of patients, and an improvement in quality of life in 76%. The median response was 8.4 months, with an overall survival of 19 months. This study confirmed the prognostic value of response rates where, at 18 months, 64% of the responders are alive versus 35% of the non-responders. This concept was recently confirmed in a retrospective analysis of the interrelationship of changes in serum PSA, palliative response and survival after systemic treatment, in a Canadian randomised trial for symptomatic hormone-refractory prostate cancer (Dowling et al. 2001). The investigators concluded that there was significant association between PSA response and palliative response. PSA response was associated with longer survival. Patients treated with mitoxantrone and prednisolone were more likely to achieve a PSA response and a palliative response than those treated with prednisolone alone.

Docetaxel has recently been used in a number of trials as a single agent to determine whether it has activity in hormone-refractory prostate cancer. Weekly administration of lower doses of docetaxel demonstrated less grade 3/4 neutropenia than was seen with the traditional 21-day cycle, making it a promising option for elderly patients or those with a poor performance status (Hainsworth et al. 1998; Burstein et al. 2000). The PSA response (> 50% decline in PSA) quoted by Picus and Schultz (1999) was 46% and the ORR was 24% in a group of 35 patients treated with the 3-weekly schedule of docetaxel 75 mg/m^2. Similar PSA response rates were quoted by Berry and Rohrborough (1999) in 59 patients treated with a weekly schedule of docetaxel 36 mg/m^2 for 8 weeks (50% PSA response of 41%). Docetaxel in combination with estramustine has demonstrated PSA response rates (> 50% decline) in 60–80% of patients (Kreis et al. 1999; Petrylak et al. 1999).

Oral fluoropyrimidines are currently being extensively investigated. A number of phase II studies have demonstrated tolerability and comparable or sometimes superior response rates to fluorouracil (FU) and 5FU-containing regimens (Ono *et al.* 1999; Kuriyama *et al.* 2001; Nishimura *et al.* 2001). Capecitabine is also undergoing clinical trials in this setting.

Palliative therapy for painful metastases

Localised bone metastases are best treated by external radiotherapy. Intravenous bisphosphonates exhibit considerable activity against pain in diffuse bone lesions, act rapidly and are relatively non-toxic.

External beam radiation

This is the mainstay of therapy for localised metastases. Metastases occur in more than 85% of hormone-resistant cancers. Pain reduction has been reported in over 75% of radiotherapy-treated patients (Allen *et al.* 1976; Epstein *et al.* 1979) and some complete responses also occurred (Dearnealey *et al.* 1992). This requires a short course of irradiation, usually 20 Gy in 10 fractions over 5 days. Irradiation of large hemibody fields is also efficient in relieving pain in over 75% of cases (6 Gy for the upper half of the body and 8 Gy for the lower half), and the benefit lasted for several months. About 80% of patients responded within 48 hours (Tong *et al.* 1982).

Strontium

Patients presenting with pain in several sites require systemic radiotherapy. Historically, phosphorus-32 (^{32}P) was used in the treatment of these patients. Treatment results have consistently demonstrated a decrease of pain in 60–80% of patients (Silberstein & Williams 1985). Major problems with the use of this radioisotope were the result of the high incidence of myelosuppression, its short half-life (14.3 days), and poor differentiation between tumour and normal bone in the radiation dose distribution. In recent years, strontium-89 (^{89}Sr) has become the radionuclide of choice. This is a pure β-emitting radionuclide which follows the same pathways as calcium. After intravenous administration, it is selectively taken up by areas of high osteoblastic activity, thus preferentially depositing the radiation dose in the region of bone metastases (Crawford *et al.* 1994). At the usual dose of 30–60 μCi/kg, it induces an almost total disappearance of bone pain in 10–50% of patients and partial disappearance in about 50% of patients. It exhibits moderate haematological toxicity (grade III/IV thrombocytopenia 4–8 weeks after injection in 20% of cases), but an OS benefit has not been demonstrated yet. Strontium-89 may induce transient increase in bone pain (flare-up) within the first few days of administration in 60% of patients. However, in combination with local external beam radiotherapy, it is associated with a reduction in the biological markers that lasts throughout the half-life of ^{89}Sr (Porter 1994). Samarium-153 is a new radionuclide which, at a dose of 1 mCi/kg, induces pain relief in 62–72% of patients with no grade IV and, rarely, grade III myelosuppression (Serarini *et al.* 1998).

Bisphosphonates

These do not have anti-tumour activity and are used in situations where the usual therapies have failed. They act on osteoclastic hyper-resorption, in areas of increased bone turnover. Clodronate and pamidronate have shown some analgesic activity in cases where the usual treatments have failed (Diener 1996).

Conclusion

In the twenty-first century, orchidectomy still remains an important and very effective intervention. However, maximum androgen blockade appears to produce maximum benefits when castration is medical and the anti-androgen is non-steroidal. Whether MAB should be continuous or intermittent is still unclear.

It is, however, clear that the nature and the duration of first-line treatments such as the introduction and subsequent withdrawal of anti-androgens may interfere with second-line hormonal therapy. Chemotherapy alone or in combination still remains of limited value in the management of patients with advanced carcinoma of the prostate, who become refractory to hormonal therapies. Indeed, no randomised study has been able to demonstrate a survival advantage with chemotherapy in this setting. At the present time, there are not enough data to choose one second-line or even a third-line therapy over another. Large trials are currently under way to identify the best possible care for patients for whom quality of life is the main concern, as defined by the patients themselves.

References

Akakura K, Bruchovsky N, Goldenberg SL *et al.* (1993). Effects of intermittent androgen suppression on androgen dependant tumours. *Cancer* **71**, 2782–2790

Allen KL, Johnson TW *et al.* (1976). Effective bone palliation as related to various treatment regimens. *Cancer* **37**, 984–987

Berry W & Rohrborough T (1999). Phase II trial of single agent weekly taxotere in symptomatic, hormone refractory prostate cancer. *Proceedings of the American Society of Clinical Oncology* **18**, 335a (abstract 1290)

Berry WR, Laszlo J, Cox E *et al.* (1979). Prognostic factors in metastatic and hormonally unresponsive carcinoma of the prostate. *Cancer* **44**, 763–775

Blackledge G, Kolvenbag G, Nash A (1996). Bicalutamide: a new antiandrogen for use in combination with castration for patients with advanced prostate cancer. *Anticancer Drugs* **7**, 27–34

Burstein HD, Manola J, Younger J *et al.* (2000). Docetaxel administered on a weekly basis for metastatic breast cancer. *Journal of Clinical Oncology* **18**, 1212–1219

Byar DP & Corle DK (1988). Hormone therapy for prostate cancer: results of the Veteran's Administration Cooperative Urological Research Group Studies. *National Cancer Institute Monograph* **7**, 165–170

Catalona WJ (1994). Management of cancer of the prostate. *New England Journal of Medicine* **15**, 996–1004

Caubet JF, Tosteson TD, Dong EW *et al.* (1997). Maximum androgen blockade in advanced prostate cancer: a meta-analysis of published randomised controlled trials using non steroidal antiandrogens. *Urology* **49**, 71–78

Chodak GW (1989). Luteinising hormone-releasing hormone (LHRH) agonists for treatment of advanced prostatic carcinoma. *Urology* **33**(suppl 5), 42–44

Chodak GW, Vogelzang NJ, Caplan RJ *et al.* (1991). Independent prognostic factors in patients with metastatic (stage D2) prostate cancer. The Zoladex Study Group. *Journal of the American Medical Association* **265**, 618–621

Crawford ED, Eisenberger MA, McLeod DG *et al.* (1989). A controlled trial of leuprolide with and without flutamide in prostatic carcinoma. *New England Journal of Medicine* **321**, 419–424

Crawford ED, Kozlowski JM, Debruyne FM *et al.* (1994). The use of strontium 89 for palliation of pain from bone metastases associated with hormone-refractory prostate cancer. *Urology* **44**, 481–485

Crawford ED, Bennett CL, Stone NN *et al.* (1997a). Comparison of perspectives on prostate cancer: analysis of survey data. *Urology* **50**, 366–372

Crawford ED, Eisenberger MA, McLeod DG *et al.* (1997b). Comparison of bilateral orchidectomy with or without flutamide for the treatment of patients with stage D2 adenocarcinoma of the prostate: results of NCI intergroup study 0105 (SWOG and ECOG). *Journal of Urology* **157**, 336a

Crawford ED, Stenner J, Rosenblum M (1998). Changing concepts in hormonal therapy. *Cancer Investigation* **16**(suppl 1), 60–62

Dahllof B, Billstrom A, Cabral F *et al.* (1993). Estramustine depolymerises microtubules by binding to tubulin. *Cancer Research* **53**, 4573–4578

Daneshgari F & Crawford ED (1993). Endocrine therapy of advanced carcinoma of the prostate. *Cancer* **71**, 1089–1093

Dawson NA (1993). Treatment of progressive metastatic prostate cancer. *Oncology* **7**, 17–24

Dearnaley DP, Bayly RJ, A'Hern RP *et al.* (1992). Palliation of bone metastases in prostate cancer: hemibody irradiation or strontium 89? *Clinical Oncology* **4**, 101–107

Denis LJ, Whelan P, Carnerio De Moura JLC *et al.* (1993). Goserelin acetate and flutamide versus bilateral orchidectomy: a phase III EORTC Trial (30853). *Urology* **42**, 119–130

Diener KM (1996). Bisphosphonates for controlling pain from metastatic bone disease. *American Journal of Health Systems and Pharmacy* **53**, 1917–1927

Dowling AJ, Panzarella T, Ernst DS *et al.* (2001). A retrospective analysis of the relationship between changes in serum PSA, palliative response and survival following systemic treatment in a Canadian randomised trial for symptomatic hormone-refractory prostate cancer. *Annals of Oncology* **12**, 773–778

Eisenberger MA & Abrams JS (1988). Chemotherapy for prostatic cancer. *Seminars in Urology* **6**, 303–310

Eisenberger MA, Crawford ED, Wolf M *et al.* (1994). Prognostic factors in stage D2 prostate cancer; important implications for future trials: results of a cooperative intergroup study (INT.0036). The National Cancer Institute Intergroup Study #0036. *Seminars in Oncology* **21**, 613–619

Eisenberger MA, Sinibaldi VJ, Reyno LM *et al.* (1995). Phase I and clinical evaluation of a pharmacologically guided regimen of suramin in patients with hormone-refractory prostate cancer. *Journal of Clinical Oncology* **13**, 2174–2186

Ellerhorst JA, Tu S, Amato RJ *et al*. (1997). Phase II trial of alternating weekly chemohormone therapy for patients with androgen independent prostate cancer. *Clinics in Cancer Research* **3**, 2371–2376

Epstein LM, Stewart BH, Antunez AR *et al*. (1979). Half and total body radiation for carcinoma of the prostate. *Journal of Urology* **122**, 330–332

Farrugia D, Ansell W, Singh M *et al*. (2000). Stilboestrol plus adrenal suppression. *British Journal of Urology International* **85**, 1069–1073

Galbraith SM & Duchesne GM (1997). Androgens and prostate cancer. Biology, pathology and hormonal therapy. *European Journal of Cancer* **33**, 545–554

Grise P, Mnif A, Navarra S *et al*. (1998). Traitement par ST52 du cancer de la prostate au stade d'échappement hormonal. *Annales de Urologie (Paris)* **32**, 39–44

Hainsworth JD, Burris HA, Erland JB *et al*. (1998). Phase I trial of docetaxel administered by weekly infusion in patients with advanced refractory cancer. *Journal of Clinical Oncology* **16**, 2164–2168

Hudes G, Roth B, Loehrer P *et al*. (1997). Phase III trial of vinblastine versus vinblastine plus estramustine phosphate for metastatic hormone refractory prostate cancer (HRPC). *Proceedings of the American Society of Clinical Oncology* **16**, 316a

Huggins C & Hodges CV (1972). Studies on prostatic cancer. I. The effect of castration, of estrogen and androgen injection on serum phosphatases in metastatic carcinoma of the prostate. *CA: A Cancer Journal for Clinicians* **22**, 232–240

Kreis W, Budmar DR, Fetten J *et al*. (1999). Phase I trial of the combination of daily estramustine and intermittent docetaxel in patients with metastatic hormone refractory prostate cancer. *Annals of Oncology* **10**, 33–38

Kristiansen P, Bergquist D, Janzon L *et al*. (1988). Thromboembolic side effects of diethyl stilbestrol diphosphate in patients with prostatic carcinoma. *Urology International* **43**, 44–46

Kuriyama M, Takahashi Y, Sahashi M *et al*. (2001). Prospective and randomised comparison of combined androgen blockade versus combination with oral UFT as an initial treatment for prostate cancer. *Japanese Journal of Clinical Oncology* **31**, 18–24

Labrie F, Dupont A, Belanger A *et al*. (1982). New hormonal therapy in prostatic carcinoma: combined treatment with an LHRH agonist and an antiandrogen. *Clinical and Investigative Medicine* **5**, 267–275

Labrie, F, Dupont A, Belanger A *et al*. (1985). Combination therapy with flutamide and castration (LHRH agonist or orchiectomy) in advanced prostate cancer: a marked improvement in response and survival. *Journal of Steroid Biochemistry* **23**(5B), 833–841

Landis SH, Murray T, Bolden S *et al*. (1999). Cancer statistics. *CA: A Cancer Journal for Clinicians* **49**, 8–31

Limonta P, Dondi D, Moretti RM *et al*. (1992). Antiproliferative effects of luteinizing hormone-releasing hormone agonist on the human prostatic cancer cell line LNCaP. *Journal of Clinical Endocrinology and Metabolism* **75**, 207–212

Matzkin H & Soloway MS (1992). Response to second-line hormonal manipulation monitored by serum PSA in stage D2 prostate carcinoma. *Urology* **40**, 78–80

Matzkin H, Eber P, Todd B *et al*. (1992). Prognostic significance of changes in prostate-specific markers after endocrine treatment of stage D2 prostatic cancer. *Cancer* **70**, 2302–2309

Medical Research Council Prostate Cancer Working Party Investigators Group (1997). Immediate versus deferred treatment for advanced prostatic cancer: initial results of the Medical Research Council Trial. *British Journal of Urology* **79**, 235–246

Miller JI, Ahmann FR, Drach GW *et al.* (1992). The clinical usefulness of serum prostate specific antigen after hormonal therapy of metastatic prostate cancer. *Journal of Urology* **147**(3 Pt 2), 956–61

Morioka M, Kobayashi T, Furukawa Y *et al.* (2002). PSA in patients with hormone refractory prostate cancer treated with low dose dexamethasone. *Urology International* **68**, 10–15

Mulders PF, Dijkman GA, Fernandez P *et al.* (1990). Analysis of prognostic factors in disseminated prostatic cancer. An update. Dutch Southeastern Urological Cooperative Group. *Cancer* **65**, 2758–2761

Nishimura K, Nonomura N, Tsujimura A *et al.* (2001). Oral combination of cyclophosphamide, uracil plus tegafur and estramustine for hormone-refractory prostate cancer. *Oncology* **60**, 49–54

Office for National Statistics (1999). *Cancer Trends in England and Wales 1950–1999*. London: Office for National Statistics

Ono Y, Ohshima S, Takahashi Y *et al.* (1999). Endocrine plus uracil/tegafur therapy for prostate cancer. *Oncology* **13**(suppl 3), 120–124

Osoba D, Tannock IF, Ernst AS *et al.* (1999). Health-related quality of life in men with metastatic prostate cancer treated with prednisone alone or mitoxantrone and prednisone. *Journal of Clinical Oncology* **17**, 1654–1663

Parker SL, Tong T, Bolden S *et al.* (1996). Cancer statistics, 1996. *CA: A Cancer Journal for Clinicians* **65**, 5–27

Petrovich Z, Baert L, Bagshaw MA *et al.* (1997). Adenocarcinoma of the prostate: innovations in management. *American Journal of Clinical Oncology* **20**, 111–119

Petrylak DP, Macarthur PB, O'Connor J *et al.* (1999). Phase I trial of docetaxel with estramustine in androgen-independent prostate cancer. *Journal of Clinical Oncology* **17**, 958–967

Picus J & Schultz M (1999). Docetaxel as monotherapy in the treatment of hormone-refractory prostate cancer. *Seminars in Oncology* **26**, 14–18

Porter AT (1994). Strontium 89 (Metastron) in the treatment of prostate cancer metastatic to bone. In Murphy G, Khoury S, Chatelain A *et al.* (eds) *4th International Symposium on Recent Advances in Urological Cancer Diagnosis and Treatment*. Paris, 22–24 June, pp 368–376

Prostate Cancer Trialists' Collaborative Group (1995). Maximum androgen blockade in advanced prostate cancer: an overview of 22 randomised trials with 3283 deaths in 5710 patients. *The Lancet* **346**, 265–269

Robson M & Dawson N (1996). How is androgen-dependent metastatic prostate cancer best treated? *Hematology/Oncology Clinics of North America* **10**, 727–47

Schellhammer PF, Sharifi R, Block NL *et al.* (1997). Clinical benefits of bicalutamide compared with flutamide in combined androgen blockade for patients with advanced prostatic carcinoma: final report of a double-blind, randomized, multicenter trial. Casodex Combination Study Group. *Urology* **50**, 330–336

Scher HI (1998). Cytotoxic chemotherapy for advanced prostate cancer: does it work, and if no, how do we prove it? In Perry MC (ed.) *Educational Book, 34th Annual Meeting ASCO*. May 16–19, Los Angeles, CA, pp 356–367

Scher HI & Kelly WK (1993). Flutamide withdrawal syndrome: its impact on clinical trials in hormone-refractory prostate cancer. *Journal of Clinical Oncology* **11**, 1566–1572

Scher HI, Steineck G, Kelly WK (1995). Hormone-refractory (D3) prostate cancer: refining the concept. *Urology* **46**, 142–148

Scher H, Mazumdar M, Vlamis V *et al.* (1996). Pre-therapy prostate specific antigen (PSA) progression and survival in androgen-independent prostate cancer (AIPC). *Proceedings of the American Society of Clinical Oncology*, vol 15, abstract 651. Boston: ASCO

Serarini AN, Houston J, Resche I *et al.* (1998). Palliation of pain associated with metastatic bone cancer using samarium-153 lexidronam: a double-blind placebo-controlled clinical trial. *Journal of Clinical Oncology* **16**, 1574–1581

Silberstein EB & Williams C (1985). Strontium-89 therapy for the pain of osseous metastases. *Journal of Nuclear Medicine* **26**, 345–348

Small EJ & Vogelzang NJ (1997). Second-line hormonal therapy for advanced prostate cancer: a shifting paradigm. *Journal of Clinical Oncology* **15**, 382–388

Tannock IF, Gospodarowicz M, Meakin W *et al.* (1989). Treatment of metastatic prostate cancer patients with low dose prednisone: evaluation of pain and quality of life as pragmatic indices of response. *Journal of Clinical Oncology* **7**, 590–597

Tannock IF, Osoba D, Stockler MR *et al.* (1996). Chemotherapy with mitoxantrone plus prednisone or prednisone alone for symptomatic hormone-resistant prostate cancer: a Canadian randomized trial with palliative end points. *Journal of Clinical Oncology* **14**, 1756–1764

Taplin ME, Bubley GJ, Shuster TD *et al.* (1995). Mutation of the androgen receptor gene in metastatic androgen independent prostate cancer. *New England Journal of Medicine* **332**, 1393–1398

Tew KD & Stearns ME (1987). Hormone independent nonalkylating mechanism of cytotoxicity for estramustine. *Urology Research* **15**, 155–160

Thorpe SC, Azmatullah S, Fellow GJ *et al.* (1996). A prospective randomized study to compare goserelin acetate (Zoladex) versus cyproterone acetate (Cyprostat) versus a combination of the two in the treatment of metastatic prostatic carcinoma. *European Urology* **29**, 47–54

Tong D, Gullick L, Hendrickson FR (1982). The palliation of symptomatic osseous metastases: final results of the radiation therapy oncology group. *Cancer* **50**, 893

Veterans Administration Cooperative Urological Research Group (1967). Treatment and survival of patients with cancer of the prostate. *Surgery, Gynecology and Obstetrics* **124**, 1011–1017

Visakorpi T, Hyytinen E, Koivisto P *et al.* (1995). In vivo amplification of the androgen receptor gene and progression of human prostate cancer. *Nature Genetics* **9**, 401–405

PART 4

Clinical governance and prostatic cancer services

Chapter 10

Effectiveness and efficiency in the co-ordination of cancer unit/cancer centre interactions: defining the role of the clinical nurse specialist

Wendy Ansell

Introduction

The brief of this chapter was to define the role of the clinical nurse specialist (CNS) in the co-ordination of the cancer unit/cancer centre interactions, looking at the effectiveness and efficiency of these interactions. In order to attempt this there is a description of how these interactions work between one cancer centre and the cancer units linked with that centre, the changes in workload over recent years and some of the changes that have occurred to facilitate continuity of care. The role encompasses the care of patients with any urological malignancy, but the emphasis will be on the part of the role that pertains to men with prostate cancer.

Background

Following the Calman–Hine report (1995), which recommended the establishment of cancer centres and cancer units in order to provide uniform access to specialist care, preferably as near to the patient's home as possible, the 'outreach' clinics at two cancer units, attended by a visiting medical oncology consultant from one cancer centre, were increased. These clinics had been started in 1982. The visiting multidisciplinary team was expanded in 1996–1997 to include also a specialist registrar (SpR) and a uro-oncology CNS. The outreach clinics take place twice a month at each hospital. With increasing numbers of patient attendances the service has been expanded to include a senior lecturer based at the centre but with clinical commitments 2 days a week at the unit (which has now become part of the centre), and the visiting outpatient service has been extended to another hospital.

Organisation

The visiting team attend the cancer units, running clinics independently but concurrently with colleagues based at the units. In two units the team work with the urologists and the third is held in the radiotherapy outpatients department. This means that there is quick and easy access to cross-referral if required. For the CNS it means that it is easy to provide a link for the patients between the different teams, to ensure that continuity of care is maintained between the different specialities and to facilitate joint consultations when needed. Any of the joint patients who are inpatients on the wards may be visited during their stay, also providing the opportunity to liaise with the ward staff and to co-ordinate care.

Statistics

The number of patient attendances has increased approximately eightfold since 1996 – see Figure 10.1 for the total numbers and Figure 10.2 for the breakdown by hospital. During this time the percentage of new referrals from the cancer units has remained consistent and comprises 20–25% of the total attendance numbers. Attendances have also increased at the cancer centre.

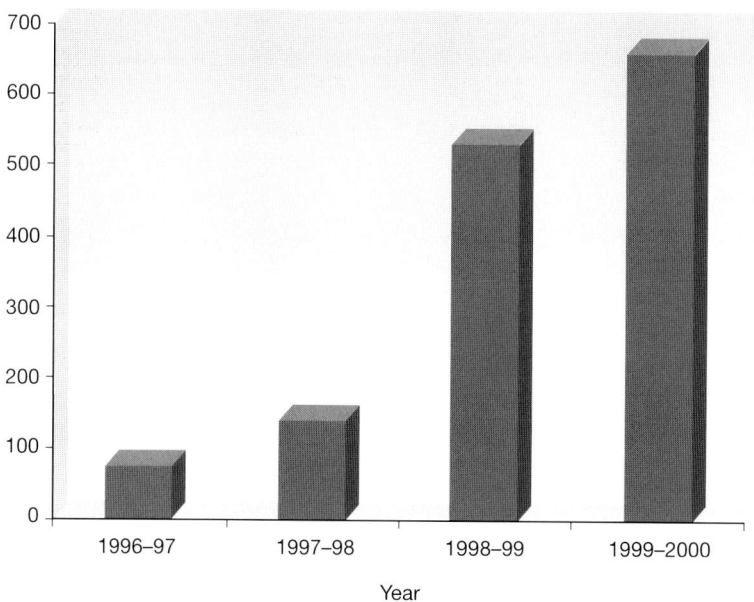

Figure 10.1 Total patient attendances at outreach clinics.

Role of the clinical nurse specialist

Although an attempt has been made by many to define the role of the CNS, there is as yet no consensus definition in the UK. The key aspects of the role of the CNS, described in detail by Chuk (1997), are the need to have clinical expertise in the speciality in order to provide direct patient care, and to be educators, consultants and researchers as part of the provision of indirect patient care – a distinction also made by Webber (1996). The overall emphasis is very much on the CNS being a part of the multidisciplinary team.

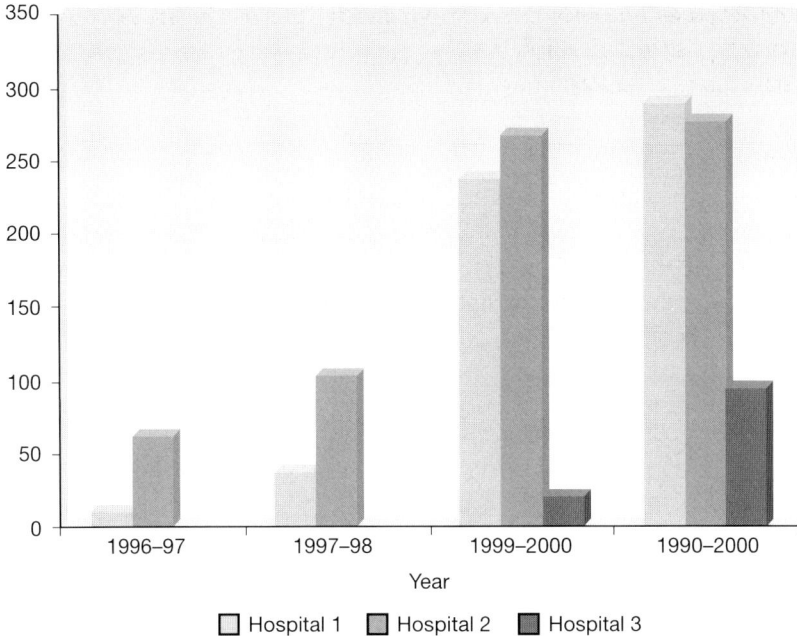

Figure 10.2 Patient attendances at outreach clinics by hospital.

Role of the uro-oncology CNS in the cancer centre/cancer unit interactions

No one job can be a blueprint for any other and the Calman–Hine report (1995) recognises that the way in which cancer networks work will vary by regions. This chapter describes the role of one CNS working in an outreach role and tries to relate this to the broader role of the CNS which is referred to non-specifically in the *NHS Cancer Plan* (Department of Health 2000a) and the *NHS Prostate Cancer Plan* (Department of Health 2000b).

Approximately 50% of patient contacts for the CNS are with people with urological malignancies attending as outpatients at the outreach clinics. This involves seeing them when they attend the clinics and remaining in contact by telephone as required. As the *NHS Cancer Plan* (Department of Health 2000a) reminds us, the largest part of any patient's cancer journey is not spent in hospital or hospice, it is spent at home and it is often when the patient is at home that their uncertainties become manifest. The telephone contact provides one way of being able to alleviate some of the anxieties before the next clinic visit is due or while tests are awaited. An audit of telephone calls made between a uro-oncology CNS and patients elsewhere (Twomey 2000) went some way to show the complexity of the role of the CNS and the amount and variety of support given through telephone calls.

At the cancer unit

At the cancer unit, the normal course of events is that the patients are seen by the consultant oncologist or the SpR. The CNS is likely to be present at the consultation of new patients or any who are known to be requiring further help or are likely to be having a change of treatment. The consultations may be 10–15 minutes for follow-up and up to 30 minutes for a new appointment, so there may have been a lot of information imparted in that time.

Following the medical consultation, the CNS may take time with the patient and their relatives/friends to go over the information they have just received if they wish. The CNS is then able to elicit how much information has been retained and understood, and the patient has the detailed knowledge of the disease and implications of potential treatment to enable them to leave the clinic with the level of understanding with which they are comfortable. It is well recognised that patients can be overwhelmed by a lot of information being imparted in a relatively short time frame and Ream (2000), in discussion of these issues, suggests that 'healthcare professionals should concentrate on providing patients with the minimum essential information and provide more detailed explanation at a later stage'. Periods of uncertainty are always difficult times and the *NHS Cancer Plan* (Department of Health 2000a) acknowledges that people want 'clear information about what is to happen at each step, and when'. This is another aspect of the clinic visit that the CNS can clarify if necessary.

According to the patients, one of the most reassuring things after they have been seen is that they have a contact number to ring if they have queries after they have had time at home to assimilate and discuss the information that they have been given. It is important to emphasise that this is not a number for emergencies and to take time to remind them of the pivotal role of their GP.

Having written information is also known to be important and newly diagnosed patients are offered the chance to take a relevant CancerBACUP booklet home with them. If they have been offered treatment on a study or have been offered chemotherapy they are also given written information to take home. If the treatment offered is a trial that is being conducted at the cancer centre, the information will have been generated at the centre and taken to the outreach clinics so there is uniformity.

At the cancer centre

On return to the cancer centre it is important that all the organisational activities are completed. The CNS may work with the medical team to ensure this occurs. The aim is to undertake the tests required at the cancer unit whenever possible, so that travelling to the centre for the patients is kept to a minimum. Some of them do need to be admitted to the centre for chemotherapy, so the team would organise this and also see them on the ward when admitted. The CNS would pass on relevant information to the ward staff such as the nursing care contacts the patient may already have, their knowledge of their disease and treatments, and any discharge planning that may have been identified already.

For some of the patients seen in the cancer unit it may have become apparent that they have symptoms not fully controlled or their illness may be progressing. At the unit, the CNS has the opportunity to elicit whether further support is needed from the community teams, and this could occur earlier in the disease pathway than it would if the CNS were not present. If permission is granted by the patient, the organisational part of this would be done back at the centre because it involves a lot of telephone communication. It may require discussion with the GP before involvement of the district nurses (DNs) and/or the community palliative care teams. This communication is very much a two-way procedure as the community teams then have a named person who knows the patient and has a wider knowledge of the specific disease and possible side effects of the treatment regimens. The community palliative care teams in particular do ring to talk through patient problems and, if necessary, following discussion with the medical 'outreach' team, appointments can easily be expedited or the doctors may ring the GP to assess the situation. These teams have expressed appreciation of this continuity of care and it provides reassurance to the patient that there is liaison between the hospital and the community staff and that they are being treated as individuals.

The Calman–Hine report(1995) highlighted the central role of the primary care team and emphasised that 'effective communication between sectors is imperative in achieving the best possible care'. *The NHS Cancer Plan* (Department of Health 2000a) has reiterated this. This is one area where the hospital-based CNS can provide a link role between the primary and secondary interface.

For men with prostate cancer

Some men who have localised prostate cancer may be referred to the medical oncologist to discuss radical treatment options if they are uncertain about radical radiotherapy or radical surgery, or they may wish to discuss newer approaches under investigation such as intermittent hormone therapy. For these men the aspect of care required from the nurse specialist at the clinic visit may be further clarification of the treatment options, help in organising their uncertainties into manageable components or ensuring that they have access to further information sources – many do make use of facilities such as the internet.

Men who have been referred to the oncologist when they have hormone-refractory prostate cancer have said that they have found it helpful to have a CNS present at the consultation and afterwards for:

* the opportunity to talk through the treatment options again;
* the opportunity to ensure they had correctly understood the information they had been given (for the reasons discussed previously);

- helping them put their disease into the context of their own life – living with their cancer;
- having a contact number – even if they do not need to use it;
- continuity of care.

The above list is anecdotal and has not been formally evaluated, and these issues are very difficult to quantify.

For the men who may be receiving novel outpatient treatments such as intermittent hormone therapy and oral chemotherapy, it does provide them with a link to the specialist who has instigated the treatment. By giving them written information about it, it also leaves them in control of their illness and treatments as much as possible. This is particularly true for those who have locally advanced or metastatic disease which is not going to be cured but with which they may be living for a number of years, and who want the best quality of life achievable. Enabling these men to live with their cancer is a very important part of the care.

One aspect of the role of the CNS is to be the first contact for the men on intermittent hormone therapy, particularly when they are 'off' treatment, so if any of their signs and symptoms recur suggesting reactivation of their disease, pre-emptive evaluation can be undertaken and their appointment brought forward. This indicates also the role of educating the patient to be in control of their disease, when and where to ring for advice, and the reassurance that there is access to the specialist advice when needed.

For the men on oral chemotherapy, the close contact with the CNS means they do not have to attend the hospital as frequently for review. Having knowledge of potential side effects and their timing and the expected outcomes of treatment means that telephone contact and support can save the men from some of the intermediary visits to outpatients.

Effectiveness and efficiency of the 'outreach' service

Effectiveness of the outreach clinics has not been formally evaluated, but the increasing numbers of attendances and the small numbers of non-attendances by patients to the clinics would suggest that the impact is a positive one. The service does provide a link between district general services and the specialist cancer centre and can reduce waiting times for access to oncologists (Farrugia & Ansell 2000). It also provides another avenue for education and support for the patients and their carers. The access to newer therapies and the opportunity to participate in clinical trials offered locally means that the patient is not denied access to these by potential difficulties in travelling to the cancer centre.

Efficiency issues, at least from the staff's viewpoint, are not all positive. It is not easy working in other hospitals and the travelling involved does take time out of the day. If patients come to clinic and are unwell, getting access to relevant help takes longer than it would at the centre purely because hospital systems are different. Ensuring that results are seen and acted upon quickly is phenomenally difficult. One of the aspects of the CNS's role in this is to provide liaison in the co-ordination of care but without spending the time doing clerical work that could be undertaken by someone else.

To take a broader outlook

Mention has been made already of the *NHS Cancer Plan* (Department of Health 2000a) which develops further the recommendations of Calman–Hine and *The NHS Prostate Cancer Programme* (Department of Health 2000b). These all make reference to the CNS as being a member of the multidisciplinary team (MDT) but in a non-specific way. There is emphasis on the importance of working as a multidisciplinary or multiprofessional team and, as part of the Cancer Services Collaborative, the *NHS Cancer Plan* quotes one team demonstrating that MDTs working together can help to reduce waiting times. *The UKCC Code of Professional Conduct* (UKCC 1992), to which each nurse is accountable, also incorporates the importance of working collaboratively with other healthcare workers, as does the Department of Health paper, *The Nursing Contribution to Cancer Care* (Department of Health 2000c).

Conclusion

Defining any role is not easy, especially when the issues veer towards qualitative ones and the CNS is only one member of a multidisciplinary team. However, the overall part of the role of the CNS with regard to the cancer unit/cancer centre interactions must be in helping to provide continuity of care in the patient's cancer journey at any time from diagnosis onwards. The continuity, communication and liaison extend across different directorates within a hospital, across trusts and across the primary/secondary and indeed tertiary interface, and aim to provide a seamless service.

Acknowledgements

The author would like to thank Professor Tim Oliver and Mr David Edwards for their advice in preparing this paper.

References

Calman K & Hine D (1995). *A Policy Framework for Commissioning Cancer Services.* London: HMSO

Chuk P Kai-Cheung (1997). Clinical nurse specialists and quality patient care. *Journal of Advanced Nursing* **26**, 501–506

Department of Health (2000a). *NHS Cancer Plan*. London: HMSO

Department of Health (2000b). *The NHS Prostate Cancer Programme*. London: HMSO

Department of Health (2000c). *The Nursing Contribution to Cancer Care*. London: HMSO

Farrugia D & Ansell W (2000). Multiprofessional care in urological cancer. *Macmillan Voice* **15**, 11–12

Ream E (2000). Information and education for patients and families. In: Kearney N, Richardson A, Fawcett-Henesy A (eds) *Cancer Nursing Practice A Textbook for the Specialist Nurse.* Edinburgh: Churchill Livingstone, pp 135–160

Twomey C (2000). Telephone contacts with a cancer nurse specialist. *Nursing Standard* **15**, 35–38

UKCC (1992). *The UKCC Code of Professional Conduct.* London: UKCC

Webber J (1996). *The Evolving Role of the Macmillan Nurse.* London: Cancer Relief Macmillan Fund

Chapter 11

Effectiveness and efficiency in clinical communication with individual patients and their carers: defining the role of the clinical nurse specialist

Heather L Gould

Introduction

Every year, approximately 15,000 men are diagnosed with prostate cancer in England and Wales. Of that number, 8,000 die. It is the second most common form of cancer in men.

With the incidence rising, there has been increasing public and government concern about how to increase early diagnosis and improve the care that these men receive. Services for patients with urological cancers and their families are very much less developed than those for other cancers, such as breast and lung. With this in mind, the big question for health professionals is: what is the best way to manage men diagnosed with prostate cancer – and their families – effectively?

With the development of the NHS Prostate Cancer Action Plan and the Calman–Hine guidelines for service provision, it is quite clear that the uro-oncology nurse specialist plays a major role in the delivery of care for the patients and family.

The role of the uro-oncology nurse specialist

> As patients' needs in hospital and home become more complex and as the care patients receive increases in sophistication, the education and knowledge of the person they turn to for help also needs to be specialised and timely.
>
> (Koetlers 1989)

In the UK, since the late 1980s, the role of the clinical nurse specialist has become well established within the core cancer team, with the breast nurse specialist becoming the foremost figure in the 1990s.

There is no single definition, but it is said that the clinical nurse specialist should be a registered nurse '… who through study and supervised practice has become an expert in a defined area of knowledge and practice on a selected clinical area of nursing …' (American Nurses Association 1980).

This remains an issue for debate and concern, as the level of practice is still not decided. The American Nurses Congress of Nursing Practice, for example, state that this should be to graduate level (masters or doctorate), although this is not the standard case in the UK. Despite the absence of an accepted definition, it is generally believed that the role of the clinical nurse specialist is complex and encompasses many subroles relating to both direct and indirect care. In essence, the role is not a universal one – each nurse works to meet the demands of his or her individual practice.

The uro-oncology nurse specialist is a relatively new concept, highlighted by the funding support from Macmillan Cancer Relief. The number of site specialist posts continues to increase across the UK. This is due to urological departments understanding such roles and being aware of the considerable benefit that they can have – not only to the core team, but also to the patient diagnosed with urological malignancy and his family.

Taking into consideration the demands of a busy uro-oncology service, the recommendations stated by the Calman–Hine report (Calman & Hine 1995) and *The Prostate Cancer Action Plan* (NHS Executive 2000), the author discusses the main aims and role of the uro-oncology nurse specialist. The author's aim in highlighting this service is to improve the effectiveness and efficiency of clinical communication between individual patients with prostate cancer and their carers.

The aim of the uro-oncology cancer service is to provide a high standard of care that takes into consideration the Calman–Hine report recommendations, which can be summarised as follows:

- All patients should have access to a uniformly high quality of care in the community or hospital wherever they may live.
- Public and professional education should be available to encourage early recognition of the symptoms of cancer.
- Patients, families and carers should be given clear information and assistance regarding treatment options and outcomes, in a form that they can understand. This should be available to them at all stages of treatment, from diagnosis onwards.
- The development of cancer services should be patient centred and take account of the views and preferences of patients, families and carers, as well as those professionals involved in cancer care.
- Access to nurse specialists with site-specific expertise should be part of the structure.

The main aims of the uro-oncology nurse specialist reflect these overall aims in the management of prostate cancer:

- To provide expert nursing advice and support to patients and their families from the time of diagnosis and through all stages of the individual cancer journey.

- To develop and monitor standards of care with the uro-oncology service and to promote education and training.
- To act as a specialist resource of up-to-date information.
- To ensure that all patients are aware of the facilities available to them within the hospital and community settings.
- To provide easy continuous access to the patients and their families.
- To provide good communication links between the hospital and community settings.

The diagnosis of prostate cancer catapults patients and their families into an unfamiliar world where they may struggle to cope with a broad range of medical, psychological and emotional issues. In order to deliver an effective and high standard of care, the uro-oncology nurse specialist should be involved at initial diagnosis. When faced with a cancer diagnosis, some patients and their families investigate and conduct extensive research using, for example, the readily available internet. This gives them a modicum of knowledge and the resultant ability to question the medical profession – in some cases to the extreme. Others adopt a much more passive 'head in the sand' approach, often to the extent that they have no wish to understand or question the diagnosis. Intervention at this point ensures that the information support required by the patients and families is provided at a correct and subjective level.

In practice
Diagnosis advisement occurs in two ways:

1 Joint uro-oncology clinic: patient access to a urologist, clinical oncologist, Macmillan uro-oncology nurse and to palliative care at one appointment. Such clinics are known to be very busy and seeing so many people following a diagnosis can be very confusing for the patients and families. Appointments can be repeated and subsequent referral to the uro-oncology nurse specialist provides a valuable link.
2 The recent development of a rapid referral clinic. This initiative is the result of the author's department working with cancer collaborative. The collaborative's main aims were to examine the current referral procedures for patients suspected to have prostate cancer and to assess the duration from referral to diagnosis: the patient journey.

  By working closely with clinical teams, the aim was to offer a faster, more streamlined service, resulting in the rapid referral clinic. Initial results show that this initiative has already speeded up the diagnosis of cancer and reduced delays for patients.

  The rapid referral clinic has been developed by the consultant and nurse specialist and aims to meet the criteria for the '2-week wait' (NHS Executive 1999). Patients with suspected prostate cancer are fast-tracked and an appointment is made. The subsequent letter to the patient informs him of the appointment and advises that it may be necessary to perform investigations. Patient information relating to the investigations is also sent out with this letter. The clinical nurse specialist meets with the patient at the first appointment and ensures that a follow-up appointment is made, usually the next week. The clinical nurse specialist is thus available at diagnosis and provides support, relevant information on treatment options, contact numbers and follow-up appointments, subject to the level of information that the patient and family wish to receive. The GP is informed at this point of the diagnosis of the proposed investigation or treatment required.

Auditing of the service suggests that the concept is proving very successful and the collaborative anticipates that this initiative will be rolled out within the local cancer services.

Both processes allow the uro-oncology nurse specialist to be involved at diagnosis and provide that essential link at a very early stage of the cancer journey. Each patient is given a card with contact numbers, together with a hand-held record card which provides the names of the clinical staff seen by the patient, a summary of what was said, the investigations required and further follow-up appointments. Each patient is encouraged to call at any time to discuss any issues or questions that may arise.

Ongoing support

Telephone support is seen as a major role of the clinical nurse specialist, with telephone helplines also being in large demand. The uro-oncology nurse specialist is well placed to be a source of contact for the patient and family. Twoomy (2000) shows, through very recent research, that telephone contact is an essential part of the clinical nurse specialist role. His research provides valuable information into the nature of telephone work within the role of the uro-oncology nurse specialist, and demonstrates the diversity of the role and the ability to provide support and information by the use of telephone contact. For example, open access patients and their families are reassured by the continuity of the care that can be delivered through a telephone support service. The growth in nurse telephone consultation services has prompted the Royal College of Nursing (1999) to produce guidelines for best practice.

Within the author's service provision it became obvious that there was the potential to incorporate a nurse-led clinic. This is a concept that has been part of the service for 2 years and is seen by the patients, urologists and community staff as an essential component in the delivery of the standard of care that prostate cancer requires. It is known that nurse-led clinics can offer a multitude of services and there is immense scope in the development of such initiatives (Poole 1996).

The main aim of the nurse-led clinic is to offer appointments away from the busy medically run clinics, and to provide valuable time, support and information in a timely, relaxed manner. After initial appointments of diagnosis, little of the information given is retained and many questions arise. The clinic provides the environment for open discussion and reassurance.

Initially, one clinic provided 4-hourly sessions. This has been increased to two clinics, one for new appointments (three slots) and another for follow-up (four slots). Referral to the clinics can be made from the consultant, oncologist, GP or the patient and family themselves.

The nurse-led clinic incorporates the following:

- General discussion and reassurance relating to the diagnosis of prostate cancer. This provides time for the patients and families to discuss their concerns and anxieties with the clinical nurse specialist, as questions do not always arise at the time of consultation.
- Discussion aimed at providing the patient with an understanding of the different treatment options available and the relative side effects of each treatment. This gives the patient valuable information and knowledge, allowing him to make an informed decision as to the preferred treatment. Not all patients necessarily want to make this choice, but it is seen that the process of decision-making increases the patients' control on the future of their disease management.
- The ongoing provision of detailed information. The nature of the information supplied obviously depends on the stage of the disease at diagnosis and, therefore, the treatment options available. It is an essential component of the uro-oncology nurse specialist to provide detailed written and verbal information relating to the specific treatment that an individual patient will receive.
- The provision of the contact details of relevant support groups and helplines – depending upon the stage of the disease and location of the patient and family. The main ones are the Prostate Cancer Support Association (0845 6010766), Macmillan Cancer Relief Information Line (0845 6016161) and CancerBACUP (020 7696 9000).
- Commencing hormone therapy: Higgins (2000) discussed this and commented that some patients who had not attended the nurse-led clinic before hormone therapy treatment worried unnecessarily about certain common side effects as they were either not discussed or not retained at initial diagnosis.
- Pre- and postoperative management of patients undergoing radical prostatectomy. The nurse-led clinic provides a valuable link for the patient with regard to the assessment of recovery and the management of incontinence and impotence, as well as referrals to other professional as required.
- New symptoms – the nurse-led clinic provides quick access back into the hospital setting for assessment and investigation of any new symptoms that the patient may have, or discussion and reassurance in relation to any new symptom that they may be worried about. If medical intervention is required, then either an appointment can be made urgently or the case referred onto the speciality required, such as a hospice or oncology opinion.

Current feedback of the clinic is good and it is considered to be a time-effective way of providing continuity of quality care.

The role of the uro-oncology nurse continues to evolve and auditing of this service is required to ensure that the patients' needs continue to be met. A review of the service's records reveals that, in the period from 1 January 2000 to 31 October 2000, 73 patients have been referred to the clinic with a diagnosis of prostate cancer, with the level of intervention varying from patient to patient; 86 appointments have been made at the clinic, some of which are repeat visits; the auditing of random days would provide valuable information on the amount of time spent on telephone contact, and the nature and number of issued addressed on the telephone.

Conclusion

Prostate cancer – its incidence, mortality rates and the cancer journey – is an area of great concern for the public, media and Government alike. The development of *The Prostate Cancer Action Plan* and the involvement of prostate cancer within the cancer collaborative poses important questions for health professionals.

The role of the clinical nurse specialists within cancer services is already well established, particularly within the fields of breast and lung cancer and as a result of the support and recognition of the benefits of such posts by Macmillan Cancer Relief.

The role of the uro-oncology nurse specialist is relatively new, but has already proved to be a valuable member of the core care team for patients diagnosed with prostate cancer and their families.

The main aim of the uro-oncology nurse specialist is to provide timely support and information from diagnosis and through the cancer journey. This is achieved by initiatives such as availability at diagnosis, telephone contacts and the provision of a nurse-led clinic.

Such initiatives have provided continuity and a prolonged contact that is essential for the treatment of prostate cancer.

The uro-oncology nurse specialist plays a major role in the overall management of the patient diagnosed with prostate cancer and his family. The role itself must become more widely available to patients and initiatives that make maximum use of that role must continue to be adopted to ensure that the overall standard of care that is provided continues to improve.

References

American Nurses Association (1980). *Nursing: A Social Policy Statement*. Kansas City, MO: ANA

Calman K & Hine F (1995). *A Policy Framework For Commissioning Cancer Services*. London: HMSO

Higgins D (2000). The role of the prostate cancer nurse specialist. *Professional Nurse* **15**, 539–542

Koetlers T (1989). Clinical practice and direct patient care. In: Hamnc A & Spross J (eds) *The Clinical Nurse Specialist in Theory and Practice,* 2nd ed. London: WB Saunders

NHS Executive (1999). *Cancer Waiting Times: Achieving the two week target.* London: NHSE

NHS Executive (2000). *The Prostate Cancer Action Plan.* London: Department of Health

Poole K (1996). The evolving role of the clinical nurse specialist within the comprehensive breast cancer centre. *Journal of Clinical Nursing* **6**, 341–349

Royal College of Nursing (1999). *Nurse Telephone Consultation Services: Information and good practice.* London: RCN Publications

Twoomy C (2000). Telephone contacts with a cancer nurse specialist. *Nursing Standard* **15**, 35–38

Health economic evaluation and cost-effectiveness of prostate cancer services: a review of current data of relevance to clinical practice and service provision

Anup Patel, Edward Rowe and Jyoti Shah

Introduction

Prostate cancer poses a major public health problem in the developed world. It is now the most commonly diagnosed male cancer (179,300 new cases in the USA in 1999, with an estimated 37,000 deaths in the same year – Landis *et al.* 1999), and the second leading cause of male cancer death after lung cancer. Prostate cancer presents a unique conundrum among human cancers with respect to issues of lead and length time bias, which stem largely from its slow tumour doubling time compared with other human epithelial tumours such as breast cancer. Indeed many men will die with an insignificant cancer (small in volume and low in grade) which will not have proved to be fatal to the host. These facts have led to an intense worldwide debate regarding the appropriateness of implementing mass screening strategies, as well as a search for the most cost-effective optimal management options if localised disease were found through screening.

During the last decade, the 'epidemic' rise in the incidence of prostate cancer in much of the developed world can be attributed to several factors. These include increased public awareness, better preventive health-seeking behaviour, an increasing ageing population, the fall in mortality from other diseases (e.g. infectious disease), but, perhaps most significantly, a steady rise in the diagnostic use of prostate-specific antigen (PSA), since the FDA (Food and Drug Administration) approved its use for this purpose in 1986. In the decade of the 1990s, this led to a steady rise in the detection of localised and thus potentially curable prostate cancer, and a decline in detection of cancer that was already advanced at diagnosis (Demers *et al.* 1994; Stamey *et al.* 1998). However, this changing pattern of disease was not without considerable financial expenditure in the USA, and yet there has been no convincing decline in prostate cancer disease specific mortality thus far.

Cost calculations and projections in health care are notoriously difficult to define due to institutional and regional variations in structure and provision of care, variation in inflationary pressures, and variations in the consumer price index for health and personal care, especially in multiple third party payer systems. In addition to the actual costs of diagnosis and delivering treatment, there are also direct non-medical costs accrued to the patient from intangible sources. These include daily transportation costs lasting 6–7 weeks for treatments such as external beam radiation, indirect costs incurred from loss of income or productivity during treatment and recovery, and costs from loss of quality of life through pain, suffering and mental anxiety. Costs also change through technical evolution of treatments, with efficient delivery of treatment and development of expertise within institutions. Various different methodologies can be used in health economics (Table 12.1), but a comprehensive discussion of these is beyond the scope of this chapter.

Table 12.1 Methods of estimating healthcare costs

Cost minimisation
Cost per case vs overall cost
Cost–utility
Cost–benefit
Cost vs charges
Cost-effectiveness
Future cost estimation (Markov modelling)

In this chapter, the current level of information available on the financial burden presented to healthcare systems by diagnosis and management of prostate cancer in all its stages is reviewed. Furthermore, the chapter aims to provide some insight into avenues of future progress in optimising service provision, balancing this with the imperative to gain the best outcomes from available resources and make provision for appropriate resource allocation in the next decade for this, the most important of male cancers.

Costs of prostate cancer screening and early detection

The issue of screening for prostate cancer is perhaps the greatest area of controversy in urological oncology at present. The rationale for screening is to increase the detection of curable prostate cancer and implement curative treatments, thereby avoiding the high cost of treating advanced disease. In rank order, the three most important factors in determining overall cost per patient screened are the *specificity* of a screening test, the *cost differential* between treatment of localised versus advanced disease and the *disease prevalence*. Presently, the most commonly available diagnostic modalities for the early detection of prostate cancer include PSA testing, digital rectal examination (DRE) and transrectal ultrasonography (TRUS) combined with prostate needle biopsy. Of these, DRE is perhaps the most commonly used in the primary care arena (Perkins *et al.* 1998). It is, however, poorly taught at medical school (Hennigan *et al.* 1991) and, in postgraduate education, is largely subjective (especially among non-urologists) and has poor sensitivity for curable disease (Catalona *et al.* 1994).

Adding DRE to PSA testing in a screening programme has a small impact on the cost per cancer detected (about a 7% increase) by almost doubling the cancer detection rate from 2.4% to 4.6%, but increasing the cost per person screened by 98% from about $US2,200 to about $US4,100. In other studies comparing the use of DRE and/or PSA, the use of DRE alone would have missed 45–50% of the cancers, compared with 10–18% that would have been missed if PSA testing alone was used. With use of both modalities, prostate cancer detection was much higher (Catalona *et al.* 1994; Candas *et al.* 2000). Furthermore, palpable cancers that are detected by DRE alone are less likely to be organ confined than those detected by PSA-based screening programmes.

In marked contrast, PSA testing involves a simple blood test and fulfils most if not all of the Wilson and Jungner (1968) criteria for a screening test. The main problem with the clinical utility of PSA testing stems from the arbitrary setting of the upper limit of normal at 4 ng/ml. Although this cut-off meant that up to 25% of early and potentially curable prostate cancer might be missed, the counterbalancing argument was that cancers producing low amounts of PSA were largely insignificant cancers unlikely to be fatal to the host. With the benefit of hindsight, this may not be the case and, consequently, biopsy thresholds in some screening programmes have been reduced to 3.5 and 3 ng/ml both in Europe and North America. The most important limitation of PSA testing has been its poor specificity in the 4–10 ng/ml range where cancers are likely to be significant and optimally curable. However, considerable expenditure and morbidity is risked from the increased requirement for TRUS-guided biopsies when the PSA is in this range.

In order to improve the specificity of PSA testing and reduce unnecessary biopsies (leading to potential cost saving), many strategies have been tried. Some of these are cheap and include the use of age- or race-specific reference ranges (which cost nothing), whereas others are expensive because they involve a hospital visit and the use of TRUS measurements (PSA density and transition zone density). More recently, refinement of the specificity of PSA testing has been made available for a little extra cost (about $US50 per test compared with about $US30 per test), by measuring the ratio of free to total PSA in serum (Catalona *et al.* 1998). In the 'grey zone' of total PSA 4–10 ng/ml, using a free-total PSA ratio cut-off of 25% would detect 95% of cancers while eliminating the need for biopsy in 20% of men with benign disease. Another factor that may have limited the specificity of PSA testing in screening programmes may be the 'miss rate' of the standard sextant biopsy technique (which ranges about 30%) (Naughton *et al.* 1998, 2000; Presti *et al.* 2000). This may be overcome in future studies by the implementation of tailored biopsy strategies based on prostate volumes (assuming that these do not lead to greater costs of processing biopsy material or a higher complication rate), because it is the larger prostate that presents the greatest diagnostic challenge. Furthermore, by lowering the upper age limit for groups eligible for cost-effective screening pilot programmes, the confounding effect of age-related increase in prostate volume should be minimised.

Two large, prospectively randomised, prostate cancer screening trials started in 1994 are currently under way in the USA and in Europe (the PLCO and the ERSPC studies). The results of these will not be known for another decade and, until then, a large disparity between the excellent diagnostic ability of PSA with an absence of discernible reduction in mortality remains to be explained. Perhaps part of the explanation stems from an observation in Michigan that the decline in prostate cancer incidence following a peak in 1992 predominantly occurred in older (>70 years) white men subject to competing mortality. Older men are a very important source of interesting management and ethical challenges as far as prostate cancer screening is concerned, but are also a source of greater cost expenditure. They are more likely to suffer harm and have worse clinical outcomes from potentially curative local therapies. Furthermore, studies from Scandinavia have shown that older men with clinically localised prostate cancer suffered only 10% disease-specific mortality compared with 66% mortality rate from competing causes (Johansson *et al.* 1992). Several other authors (Fleming *et al.* 1993; Beck *et al.* 1994; Kattan *et al.* 1997; Albertsen *et al.* 2000) have emphasised the impact of grade on survival. They have demonstrated that older men only stand to gain from any active treatment for prostate cancer compared to observation if they have moderate or poorly differentiated tumours, or if they are likely to survive at least 10 more years than their present age. Consequently it seems intuitive that early detection efforts in men who are 70 years of age or older have marginal benefit in a cost-effectiveness ratio analysis even under favourable circumstances, as demonstrated by Coley *et al.* (1997). From a cost-effectiveness perspective, there should be a trend towards dissuading elderly men from inclusion in mass screening programmes, and towards advocating less aggressive local therapy or no immediate therapy in the elderly cohort with well or moderately differentiated localised disease.

In general, large-scale unrestricted screening studies are expensive, involve the recruitment of large numbers of men and may be obsolete by the time the results are known. The comparative cost implications on screening for prostate cancer show that screening programmes that implement serial screening episodes are more cost-effective than those using a single screening episode. The reason for this is the lower cancer detection rate after the first screen, which itself should pick up a large proportion of the prevalence of cancers in the first year of screening. Once these have been detected, future cancers will decrease to the incidence level of the disease. Serial screening should therefore identify a greater proportion of organ-confined cancers after the first year. In this case, fewer diagnostic and staging tests should be required and local treatment should have a better cure rate with a reduced requirement for extra expenditure in local salvage therapies or in treating distant progression, all of which would offset the higher initial cost of serially detected cancers. Moreover, less expenditure should be incurred, as compliance with serial screening tends to decline except in motivated patients keen to avoid the consequences of advanced disease.

Littrup (1997) compared various methods for cost-effective prostate cancer detection (Table 12.2) and found that use of age-related PSA thresholds and a tailored biopsy strategy gave the best positive predictive value (33.8%) and the lowest cost per cancer detected ($US3,144). Use of a tailored biopsy approach itself, irrespective of PSA, could translate into an annual saving of $US67 million in the USA (provided the cost of processing tailored biopsy material did not increase prohibitively). They emphasised that relative cancer risk, clinical ease of use and cost-efficacy should dominate the selection of cancer detection strategies. This study pre-dated the era of improvements in the specificity performance of PSA testing using free total PSA ratios, which in itself has the potential to eliminate unnecessary prostate needle biopsies without loss of sensitivity and without incurring costs from TRUS (Catalona *et al.* 1998).

Table 12.2 Cost-effectiveness of different prostate cancer detection approaches for screening

Screen strategy	Biopsy strategy	Screen +ve (%)	Cancer +ve (%)	PPV	Biopsy cost ($US)	Cost/ cancer ($US)
Age PSA	Tailored	12	3.2	33.8	49,000	3,144
Age PSA	Systematic	12	3.3	28.8	60,000	3,382
PSA 4 alone	Tailored	15.6	3.4	30.8	58,000	3,414
PSA 3 alone	Tailored	22.7	3.7	29.7	64,000	3,645
Age PSA & DRE	Tailored	21.4	3.9	27.4	74,000	4,259
PSA 4 & DRE	Tailored	24.4	4.1	28.1	80,500	4,320
DRE alone	Tailored	12.4	2.5	21.2	62,000	4,511
PSA 4 & DRE	Systematic	24.4	4.6	19.5	122,000	4,752

PPV, positive predictive value.

Unfortunately, the ideal serial screening interval is not yet known, and may be anywhere from 1 to 3 years. At present, it can only be estimated by statistical modelling using tools such as log linear regression analyses and Markov models (Ross *et al.* 2000). The risks of screening are faced upfront, whereas the potential benefits in terms of longevity (approximately 3 years of life for a cancer detected at age 55 years and 1.5 years for one detected at 65 years of age) will not be realised for a decade or more. Therefore, efficient and impartial counselling and 'informed consent' using written and videotape material on relative cancer risk versus benefit, or lack thereof, becomes more important before any screening takes place. However, this has never been implemented in any large-scale screening study to date.

If there is no consensus on mass screening of the 'worried well' to detect sporadic prostate cancer on a cost-effectiveness rating, there can be little doubt that the prospect for reducing mortality is highest in those with the highest prevalence for prostate cancer, and in those with more biologically aggressive tumours where the likelihood of progression increases. Thus the targeting of high-risk groups for regular testing with a blood test that has the best specificity without significant loss of sensitivity makes more socioeconomic sense, particularly when investing limited screening resources for the maximum potential gain. Such a strategy could easily be piloted in those with a 10-year life expectancy and either a familial history of prostate cancer (10% of all prostate cancer incidence) or an African–Caribbean racial origin, both in the UK and the USA. These groups of men are most likely to have more biopsy cores with cancer and more cores containing any cancer of Gleason score ≥4. Furthermore, screening with a blood test alone is more likely to be acceptable among black men than a strategy that includes DRE, due to different cultural attitudes to DRE in this cohort, compounded by an overall distrust and fear of cancer-related issues in general.

Transrectal ultrasonography, although now widely available, is expensive and rarely performed by trained urologists, and many studies have confirmed its lack of sensitivity and specificity for the detection of curable early prostate cancer. Despite the fact that hypoechoic lesions on TRUS are more likely to contain cancer, up to 50% of cancers would be missed if only these areas were biopsied (Ellis *et al.* 1994). Moreover, like any other imaging modality currently available, it has severe limitations in detecting microscopic local invasion especially in clinical T2 disease. It is a good way of targeting biopsies when the approach is tailored and can be used for PSA density calculations (although this may be subject to observer variation and interobserver errors). It is, however, very expensive ($US6,520 per cancer versus $US2,205 for PSA alone, or $US4,108 for DRE alone) as a screening test and not particularly sensitive or specific. It should not be used as part of a screening strategy in the way that is analogous to mammography in breast cancer screening.

Comparative costs of early detection of prostate cancer

Perhaps the greatest controversy in urological oncology presently is the issue of screening for early detection of prostate cancer. If effective, screening should reduce the number of cases of advanced prostate cancer and hence the associated costs. The cost of managing advanced prostate cancer has been averaged at $US11,182 per patient in one European study (Beemsterboer *et al.* 1999), and in some North American estimates it is as high as $US35,000–100,000, compared to the cost of local treatment which is approximately $US20,000–30,000.

Breast cancer screening is currently routinely available to women in the UK. As with prostate cancer, the major cost saving for breast cancer screening is made through the prevention of advanced disease. Approximately 40% of the extra costs due to the breast cancer-screening programme were compensated for by the prevention of the advanced stage (Beemsterboer *et al.* 1999). This compares to a 10% saving with cervical cancer screening programs. Many other comparisons have been made between existing screening programmes such as those for breast cancer screening and PSA testing for the prostate. A man over 50 years with an abnormal PSA level is twice as likely to have a cancer than a woman over the age of 50 years with an abnormal mammogram (Kerlikowska *et al.* 1993). PSA appears to have a tenfold greater detection rate than mammography for two diseases that have similar incidence and mortality rates (Littrup 1997). There has been little difference in studies looking at the economic burden for prostate cancer screening compared with breast cancer screening. Benoit and Naslund (1994) estimated the screening cost per carcinoma detected at $US2,372 for 50- to 69-year-old men compared to $US10,975 per breast carcinoma detected by screening. Furthermore, breast cancer screening also detects clinically insignificant DCIS (ductal carcinoma *in situ*) at a rate of 15–40% in screening programmes and up to 50–70% of this will remain latent. Hence, the latent cancer detection rate for both breast and prostate cancer are similar and are unlikely to change the relationship between the two in screening cost terms.

In summary, screening for breast cancer has been widely accepted in the UK and has been the subject of many public awareness campaigns and fundraising efforts from the participation of the show business and fashion industries, whereas screening for prostate cancer has not. Yet it can be rightly argued that breast cancer screening is 3.7–5.2 times more costly, and has a lower cancer detection rate (0.65–1.3% versus 2.5–4.6%) compared to prostate cancer screening. Both diseases have similar long-term survival characteristics for organ-confined disease. Current data seem to suggest that breast cancer screening reduces mortality in women older than 50 years by up to 30%, and in order to achieve equivalence, only a 6–8% reduction in mortality of prostate cancer would be required through a screening programme, an easily achievable target.

Costs of staging prostate cancer

Once prostate cancer has been diagnosed, it is vital to evaluate the extent of tumour extension. There are, however, no guidelines or consensus on which, if any, imaging modality to use in this staging process. The percentage of screen-detected cancers that are both significant and curable has dramatically increased, and should potentially lead to savings from unnecessary staging investigations, and yet money is still wasted performing these as a matter of routine.

Computed tomography (CT) is popular, costs $US400–800 and is now readily available in most UK hospitals, but appears to have very limited use in prostate cancer staging. In one study from the US, all 244 patients with a PSA of < 15, clinical stage of cancer less than T2b and Gleason sum < 7 had negative CT scans (Lee *et al.* 1999). Others have sensibly recommended that CT scans should be reserved only for men at high risk of identifiable nodal metastases. Wolf *et al.* (1995) calculated that an astonishing $US50,661 would need to be spent per man to avoid an unnecessary radical prostatectomy for node-positive disease if all men routinely had a pelvic CT or magnetic resonance imaging (MRI).

The value of routine radio-isotope bone scanning in all newly diagnosed prostate cancer patients has also been questioned and shown to be unnecessary. In a study of 3,600 men with prostate cancer, there was a low positive yield using bone scans (Table 12.3). This has been confirmed by others (Lin *et al.* 1999) in patients with low PSA levels (<50 ng/ml) and Gleason Sum Scores <6 (Table 12.4). Looking at all men with positive bone scans, the median PSA was found to be 158 ng/ml. Yet in a survey of clinical practice sponsored by the American Urological Association (AUA), 40% of American urologists routinely used this test in working up men with localised prostate cancer (Gee *et al.* 1995; Barry *et al.* 1997). Avoiding bone scans on men with a PSA < 15 ng/ml would lead to a saving of $US38 million per annum.

Table 12.3 The positive yield for bone scans and CT scans

	PSA 4–20 (%)	Gleason sum < 6 (%)	PSA > 50 or Gleason sum 8–10 & PSA>20 (%)
Positive bone scan	< 5	2	>10
Positive CT scan	<12	9	>20

Albertsen *et al.* 2000.

Table 12.4 Number of positive bone scans based on PSA value and Gleason sum

PSA value	Positive bone scan
10.1 – 20	2/34 (6%)
20.1 – 50	3/29 (10%)
>50.1	16/30 (53%)

Gleason sum	Positive bone scan
< 6	4/160 (2.5%)
> 7	20/110 (18%)

Another frequently used modality is MRI. It too is hampered by its inability to reliably detect microscopic spread or nodal disease in well/moderately differentiated tumours of Gleason grade 2–6 and PSA < 20 and its high cost precludes its routine application (Rifkin *et al.* 1990). Its only real value is in detecting seminal vesical invasion (assuming that this knowledge would influence treatment choice) or in looking at bone structure for metastatic disease when bone scans and plain radiographs are suspicious but inconclusive.

Treatment of localised prostate cancer

Radical prostatectomy, either perineal or retropubic is often referred to as the current gold standard, with almost 95% of urologists in the USA recommending this treatment option to those aged 70 years or less with organ-confined disease

(Drachenberg 2000). Radical prostatectomy arguably has the best cure rates for organ-confined prostate cancer, but at significant cost. In fact, radical retropubic prostatectomy accounts for just under half of all prostate cancer costs in the USA ($US841 million). Much of these costs are faced immediately, with long inpatient hospital stays (average 5–10 days), blood transfusion (and autologous donations in some countries), the need to wear a catheter for 2 weeks postoperatively and use of incontinence pads for anywhere up to a year or more. Added to these are costs of managing treatment-related complications. These include managing positive margins (a 40% margin positive rate in some of the 'best' series in the UK) requiring salvage external beam radiation cost, treatment of impotence (much higher outside a handful of 'centres of excellence' in the USA) and urinary incontinence (including the cost of further surgery such as the implantation of an artificial urethral sphincter). Other complications include managing anastomotic strictures, lymphoceles and treatment of thromboembolic problems. Furthermore, there is a cost to the individual in terms of loss of income for an average period of 6 weeks, not to mention intangible losses from restriction of activities until continence and potency are regained in those with good outcomes.

Hospital costs associated with radical prostatectomy have been reduced in the past 5 years or so by the realisation that home bowel preparation, avoiding opiate analgesia in favour of long-acting non-steroidal analgesia, and implementation of multidisciplinary integrated care pathways (ICP), could lead to significant savings. In a study from UCLA, Litwin *et al.* (1996) showed that the use of an ICP led to a 12% reduction in hospital costs (from $US7,916 to $US6,934), a larger reduction in hospital charges from $US17,005 to $US13,524 and a 28% reduction in hospital stay from 5 to 3.6 days. Although operating room costs were unaffected by such measures, institutional costs from elimination of unnecessary radiology costs (–73%), lab tests (–47%), medical and surgical supply (–36%), room and nursing care cost (–29%) and pharmacy costs (–19%) accounted for the majority of the savings.

Changing the surgical approach to perineal prostatectomy may also shorten hospital stay and transfusion requirement. However, this is not widely available and may be disadvantaged by higher margin-positive rates, an inability to perform simultaneous nodal staging where appropriate, and lower potency rates. It is too soon to know the cost impact of the newly developed technique of laparoscopic radical prostatectomy. In the short term, it is likely to be expensive in terms of operating room cost (especially from the high cost of disposable equipment) and this can only be partially offset by the shorter hospital stay and an earlier return to work (neither of which have yet been proven).

The alternative to curative surgery is attempted cure with organ, and therefore functional preservation, using radiotherapy (either standard external beam radiation, three-dimensional conformal external beam radiation [3-DCRT] with or without dose escalation, and temporary or permanent interstitial radiation brachytherapy).

In terms of cost analyses, 3-DCRT has greater initial work-up and treatment cost amounting to $US17,259 from one US centre versus $US9,800 for conventional radiotherapy (Horwitz *et al.* 1999). The authors suggested that the better efficacy of 3-DCRT for both biochemical and clinical disease control led to a narrowed cost differential between the two treatments with time and that, after 8 years, the mean total charge was less for the 3-DCRT group ($US8,955.48 versus $US10,544.53). This difference did not reach statistical significance. Other studies (Cho *et al.* 1999) have found no difference between the two types of treatment at the same dose level, and have suggested that more evidence is needed on the improved longer-term efficacy of 3-DCRT at the higher dose level. Thus the two treatments may be equivalent in costs, only provided there is no excess late morbidity with 3-DCRT ± dose escalation when such treatments are disseminated for widespread consumption/delivery beyond a few centres of excellence. The costs of external beam radiation are also escalating as recent studies begin to show statistically significant improvements in survival benefit when radiation is combined with extended periods of neoadjuvant and adjuvant hormonal therapy with expensive gonadotrophin-releasing hormone (GnRH) analogues (Bolla *et al.* 1997; Roach *et al.* 2000).

Transperineal prostate brachytherapy with permanent implantation of radioactive iodine or palladium seeds is the latest modern iteration of interstitial radiation for the curative treatment of localised prostate cancer. The long-term efficacy of this treatment is not widely known outside a handful of centres in the USA. Nevertheless it has rapidly become popular as patients are attracted to its minimal invasiveness, reduced inpatient hospitalisation and lower morbidity, certainly with respect to urinary incontinence and possibly with regard to impotence. Other perceived advantages are higher overall radiation dose compared with that which can be achieved by external beam techniques, albeit at a lower dose rate. In the UK, prostate brachytherapy is not as yet widely available, and there is no provision for the treatment to be funded by the National Health Service even as part of a New Health Technologies Assessment. Moreover, the use of palladium-103 (which has a shorter half-life than iodine-125) is heavily restricted by UK radiation licensing authorities. Several studies from individual institutions have recently compared charges of brachytherapy to surgery (Table 12.5), and most of these show a slightly higher cost for brachytherapy, notwithstanding the cost of treating complications for either treatment. Close scrutiny of these costs show that the excess cost of brachytherapy stems mainly from the cost of the isotope (Ciezki *et al.* 2000), higher professional costs (as the procedure is performed by a team that includes a radiation oncologist, a urologist or uro-radiologist and a physicist), and the cost of extra radiology such as post-implant CT scans to determine dose volume histograms for quality assurance assessments. Palladium-103 is also more expensive than iodine-125. All other costs substantially favour brachytherapy. The cost of seeds will remain high until competition in the number of isotope suppliers increases and serves to reduce the cost, but this fall will largely be driven by an increase in the number of brachytherapy procedures. The end-result may be an increase in overall brachytherapy expenditure if more localised disease is found through greater utility of PSA-based early detection, and if demand for the treatment is driven by patient preference. Various strategies have been proposed to drive down the cost per procedure for prostate brachytherapy. One study has suggested the use of fewer higher activity seeds implanted with a peripheral loading plan, which is significantly cheaper than techniques using lower strength seeds and more uniform loading. At current prices, treatment plans using peripheral loading with 0.75 mCi/seed yielded an approximate 55% savings in total seed cost compared to plans using the most commonly ordered 0.34 mCi seed, but such a strategy leaves little technical margin for error as fewer high activity seeds are implanted. Long-term results are therefore needed to confirm efficacy and toxicity of use of such variations in seed activities (Maguire *et al.* 2000). Another approach is to perform both the planning study and the implant in a single sitting (real-time planning), although this requires a high institutional throughput of patients. Only then can enough isotope be preordered and kept on site to be used in time to avoid loss of efficacy through decay in radioactivity. One thing is clear, that brachytherapy is here to stay for now at least as a result of increasing patient interest and the willingness to pay in those with appropriate resources. A regionally based financial provision for this modality new to the UK, is therefore imperative within future planning of NHS budgets, if this modality is to be delivered cost-effectively.

Table 12.5 Comparison of relative charges: brachytherapy (BxRT) vs radical retropubic prostatectomy (RRP)

Author	Duration	BxRT charge ($US)	RRP charge ($US)	RR
Wagner *et al.* (1999)	Perioperative	21,025	15,097	1.39
Ellis (1999)	Perioperative	20,055	17,582	1.14
Optenberg & Thompson (1999)	4 months	15,261	11,910	1.28
Kohan *et al.* (1999)	1 year	14,203	14,567	0.97

RR, relative cost of BxRT to RRP (based on charges).

Offsetting the potential for cost savings, just as with external beam radiation, the indications for neoadjuvant GnRH analogues before monotherapy brachytherapy have yet to be studied prospectively. Retrospective evidence seems to suggest that it may be beneficial in improving outcomes for intermediate and high-risk patients (with respect to extraprostatic spread). Hormonal down-sizing for 3 months is mandatory for prostates larger than 50–60 cm³ to avoid pubic arch interference and enable a good quality implant. It may also reduce the incidence of the complication of acute urinary retention and avoid the need for salvage transurethral prostatectomy, which itself carries a high risk (up to 40%) of urinary incontinence. For men with prostate cancer that may already be locally advanced at diagnosis (which could represent up to one-third of all new prostate cancer cases in the UK), it may be necessary to combine an implant with a course of external beam radiation (± short-term GnRH analogues) to optimise the chance of local cure. Although this would considerably increase the immediate overall cost of treatment, if it led to better outcomes or lower morbidity than are possible with prolonged hormonal therapy in combination with 3-DCRT (with dose escalation), it may yet be cost-effective. Issues such as these must be studied from a cost-effectiveness perspective in well-designed prospectively randomised trials in the coming decade.

Treatment of advanced disease

Advanced prostate cancer treatment has a mean duration of about 24 months before cancer death, and during this time, the cost of care may range from $US11,181 to $US100,000 depending on the healthcare system concerned. In rank order, costs are accrued from inpatient stay (mean 28–35 days), control of pain, treatment of urinary problems due to local progression, treatment of malaise, treatment of neurological problems, and treatment of other associated problems. In a study from the Netherlands (Beemsterboer *et al.* 1999), 49% of the overall net cost was from hospital stay, 21% was from hormonal treatment, while palliative radiation therapy accounted for 11%. This last cost would be much higher if expensive drugs such as strontium-89 came into routine clinical use (at an approximate cost in the authors' institution of $US3,420 per treatment) to relieve bone pain from metastatic disease. Outpatient visits only accounted for 3% whereas surgical treatment (orchidectomy or TURP) accounted for only 2%.

Hormonal treatment has become increasingly expensive and has eclipsed surgical orchidectomy as the treatment of choice for advanced disease despite being more expensive in the long term (Rutqvist & Wilking 1992; Chamberlain *et al.* 1997; Bonzani *et al.* 1998). For the first time, a study (Medical Research Council Prostate Cancer Working Party Investigators Group 1997) has hinted at an advantage for early hormonal therapy versus delayed therapy. The case for widespread use of combined androgen blockade is by no means proven and when this fact is accepted in urological practice, should lead to further cost saving. This may be further augmented by the results of ongoing intermittent hormonal studies, provided disease control rates are not significantly shortened. If one considers comparative costs of treating advanced prostate and breast cancer, the duration of advanced prostate cancer is longer than breast cancer (24 vs 21 months), while prostate cancer has a shorter duration of hospital stay than breast cancer (27 v 45 days). Thus, the absolute costs are lower for prostate cancer compared with breast cancer. There are no cost data in the literature for hospice care of advanced prostate cancer compared with hospital care, but provision must be adequate for this very important component of treating any patient with terminal malignant illness during resource allocation.

Conclusion

Time trends have shown escalating costs in the incidence and treatment of prostate cancer as the post-war population balance shifts lead to a greater proportion of older men with reduced co-morbidity from other illnesses. These higher costs are a small proportion of the overall health budget for a nation with a nationalised healthcare system (estimated 0.1–1.3%) (Krahn *et al.* 1999), and stem mainly from an increase and perhaps unselective utility of PSA testing by non-specialists (Poteat *et al.* 2000). This leads to more biopsies, a greater demand for curative treatment and, at present failure rates, increased use of salvage therapy, plus higher drug costs and an increased utility of GnRH analogues (in an adjuvant and neoadjuvant setting, in maximum androgen blockade regimens, and in earlier treatment of advanced disease).

There are many economic potentials for significant cost savings. Increasing the specificity of a simple screening test (perhaps in exchange for a small loss in sensitivity in older men) should lead to fewer biopsies. Discouraging low prevalence groups from participating in screening programmes while enhancing the participation of high-risk men in targeted screening programmes (thus avoiding the high costs of treating advanced disease in this subset) will produce cost savings. Reducing the costs of staging through implementation of practice guidelines, and reducing inpatient hospital costs through adoption of validated evidence-based multidisciplinary integrated care pathways combined with the use of minimally invasive therapeutic regimens without loss of efficacy of cancer control or cure, will also serve as potentials for future cost savings. In this way, the quality of care can be maintained at a lower cost, with less individual variation and limitation of practices that are unnecessary or of marginal value (particularly those that relate to high volume or high cost laboratory or radiology tests).

This can best be achieved through the development of a comprehensive national prostate cancer network based around regional multidisciplinary reference centres backed by a supporting network of urologists and medical oncologists. These reference centres should promote local cost containment through the implementation of evidence-based practice guidelines and provide national treatment standards of best practice. They should be accessible to all men with suspected prostate cancer and should facilitate and expedite the patient cancer journey by providing one-stop diagnostic clinics run by subspecialist uro-oncologists and appropriate support staff. An appropriately funded national framework, where funding follows the patient rather than the present system where it leads the patient, is essential. It will enable the next generation of urological surgeons to be trained in appropriate TRUS biopsy techniques, in sphincter and nerve sparing but not cancer-sparing surgical techniques, and establish an appropriate setting to deliver all the treatment options for local and advanced disease in a multidisciplinary setting. It will allow the next generation of medical oncologists and allied professions to be trained in modern organ-preserving alternatives to surgery such as brachytherapy and three-dimensional conformal external beam radiation. It will also establish a broad-based platform to conduct meaningful clinical and cross-discipline translational research to optimise prostate cancer therapy across the board in the next decade and beyond.

References

Albertsen PC, Hanley JA, Harlan LC *et al.* (2000). The positive yield of imaging studies in the evaluation of men with newly diagnosed prostate cancer: a population based analysis. *Journal of Urology* **163**, 1138–1143

Barry MJ, Fowler FJ Jr, Bin L *et al.* (1997). A nation-wide survey of practising urologists: current management of benign prostatic hyperplasia and clinically localised prostate cancer. *Journal of Urology* **158**, 488–491

Beck JR, Kattan MW, Miles BJ (1994). A critique of the decision analysis for clinically localized prostate cancer. *Journal of Urology* **152**, 1894–1899

Beemsterboer PM, de Koning HJ, van der Maas PJ *et al.* (1999). Advanced prostate cancer: course, care and cost implications. *Prostate* **40**, 97–104

Benoit RM & Naslund MJ (1994). An economic rationale for prostate cancer screening. *Urology* **44**, 795–803

Bolla M, Gonzalez D, Warde P *et al.* (1997). Improved survival in patients with locally advanced prostate cancer treated with radiotherapy and gosarelin. *New England Journal of Medicine* **337**, 295–300

Bonzani RA, Stricker HJ, Peabody JO *et al.* (1998). Cost comparison of orchidectomy and leuprolide in metastatic prostate cancer. *Journal of Urology* **160**, 2446–2449

Candas B, Cusan L, Gomez JL *et al.* (2000). Evaluation of PSA and digital rectal examination as screening tests for prostate cancer. *Prostate* **45**, 19–35

Catalona WJ, Richie JP, Ahmann FR *et al.* (1994). Comparison of digital rectal examination and serum PSA in the early detection of prostate cancer: Results of a multicentre trial of 6330 men. *Journal of Urology* **157**, 1283–1290

Catalona WJ, Partin AW, Slawin KM *et al.* (1998). Use of the percentage of free prostate specific antigen to enhance differentiation of prostate cancer from benign prostate disease: a prospective multicentre clinical trial. *Journal of the American Medical Association* **279**, 1542–1547

Chamberlain J, Melia J, Moss S *et al.* (1997). Report prepared for the health technology assessment panel of NHS executive on the diagnosis, management, treatment and costs of prostate cancer in England and Wales. *British Journal of Urology* **79**, 1–32

Cho KH, Khan FM, Levitt SH (1999). Cost-benefit analyses of 3D conformal radiation therapy – treatment of prostate cancer as a model. *Acta Oncol* **38**, 603–611

Ciezki JP, Klein EA, Angermeier KW *et al.* (2000). Cost comparison of radical prostatectomy and transperineal brachytherapy for localised prostate cancer. *Urology* **55**, 68–72

Coley CM, Barry MJ, Fleming C *et al.* (1997). Early detection of prostate cancer. Part II: Estimating the risks, benefits, and costs. American College of Physicians. *Annals of Internal Medicine* **126**, 468–479

Demers RY, Swanson GM, Weiss LF (1994). Increasing incidence of cancer of the prostate. The experience of black and white men in the Detroit metropolitan area. *Archives of Internal Medicine* **154**, 1211–1216

Drachenberg DE (2000). Treatment of prostate cancer: watchful waiting, radical prostatectomy, and cryoablation. *Seminars in Surgical Oncology* **18**, 37–44

Ellis WJ (1999). Comparative single institution costs of radical prostatectomy, prostate seed implantation, and prostate seed implantation combined with external beam radiation therapy (Abstract 591). *Journal of Urology* **161**, 154

Ellis WJ, Chetner MP, Preston SD *et al.* (1994). Diagnosis of prostatic carcinoma: the yield of PSA, digital rectal examination and transrectal ultrasound. *Journal of Urology* **52**, 1520–1525

Fleming C, Wasson JH, Albertsen PC *et al.* (1993). A decision analysis of alternative treatment strategies for clinically localised prostate cancer. Prostate Patient Outcomes Research Team. *Journal of the American Medical Association* **269**, 2650–2658

Gee WF, Holtgreeve HL, Albertsen PC *et al.* (1995). Practice trends in the diagnosis and management of prostate cancer in the United States. *Journal of Urology* **154**, 207–208

Hennigan TW, Franks PJ, Hocken DB *et al.* (1991). Influence of undergraduate teaching on medical students' attitudes to rectal examination. *British Medical Journal* **302**, 829

Horwitz, Hanlon AL, Pinover WH *et al.* (1999). The cost effectiveness of 3D conformal radiation therapy compared with conventional techniques for patients with clinically localised prostate cancer. *International Journal of Radiation Oncology Biology Physics* **45**, 1219–1225

Johansson JE, Adami HO, Anderson PC *et al.* (1992). High 10-year survival rate in patients with early untreated prostate cancer. *Journal of the American Medical Association* **267**, 2191–2196

Kattan MW, Cowen ME, Miles BJ (1997). A decision analysis for treatment of clinically localized prostate cancer. *Journal of General Internal Medicine* **12**, 299–305

Kerlikowska K, Grady D, Barclay J et al. (1993). Positive predictive value of screening mammography by age and family history of breast cancer. *Journal of the American Medical Association* **270**, 2444–2450

Kohan AD, Armenakas NA, Fracchia JA (1999). Perioperative charge equivalence of radical prostatectomy and brachytherapy (Abstract 45). *Journal of Urology* **161**, 12

Krahn MD, Coombs A, Levy IG (1999). Current and projected annual direct costs of screening asymptomatic men for prostate cancer using prostate-specific antigen. *CMAJ* **160**, 49–57

Landis SH, Murray T, Bolden S *et al.* (1999). Cancer statistics, 1999. *CA: Cancer Journal for Clinicians* **49**, 8–31

Lee N, Newhouse JH, Olsson CA *et al.* (1999). Which patients with newly diagnosed prostate cancer need a computed tomography scan of abdomen and pelvis? An analysis based on 528 patients. *Urology* **54**, 490–494

Lin K, Szabo Z, Chin BB, Civelek AC (1999). The value of a baseline bone scan in patients with newly diagnosed prostate cancer. *Clinical Nuclear Medicine* **24**, 579–582

Littrup PJ (1997). Future benefits and cost effectiveness of prostate carcinoma screening. *Cancer* **80**, 1864–1870

Litwin MS, Smith RB, Thind A *et al.* (1996). Cost-efficient radical prostatectomy with a clinical care path. *Journal of Urology* **155**, 989–993

Maguire PD, Waterman FM, Draher AP (2000). Can the cost of permanent prostate implants be reduced? An argument for peripheral loading with higher strength seeds. *Techniques in Urology* **6**, 85–88

Medical Research Council Prostate Cancer Working Party Investigators Group (1997). Immediate versus deferred treatment for advanced prostatic cancer: initial results of the Medical Research Council trial. *British Journal of Urology* **79**, 235–246

Naughton CK, Smith DS, Humphrey PA *et al.* (1998). Clinical and pathologic tumour characteristics of prostate cancer as a function of the number of cores: a retrospective study. *Urology* **52**, 808–813

Naughton CK, Omstein DK, Smith *et al.* (2000). Pain and morbidity of transrectal guided ultrasound prostate biopsies: a prospective randomised trial of 6 versus 12 cores. *Journal of Urology* **163**, 168–171

Optenberg SA & Thompson I (1999). Comparative analysis of total perioperative charges of radical prostatectomy and brachytherapy (Abstract 44). *Journal of Urology* **161**, 11

Perkins JJ, Sanson-Fisher RW, Clarke SJ *et al.* (1998). An exploration of screening practices for prostate cancer and the associated community expenditure. *British Journal of Urology* **82**, 524–529

Poteat HJ, Chen P, Loughlin KR *et al.* (2000). Appropriateness of prostate-specific antigen testing. *American Journal of Clinical Pathology* **113**, 421–428

Presti JC Jr, Chang JJ, Bhargava V *et al.* (2000). The optimal systematic prostate biopsy scheme should include 8 rather than 6 biopsies: results of a prospective clinical trial. *Journal of Urology* **163**, 163–166

Rifkin MD, Zerhouni EA, Gastonis CA *et al.* (1990). Comparison of magnetic resonance imaging and ultrasonography in staging early prostate cancer. Results of a multi-institutional co-operative trial. *New England Journal of Medicine* **323**, 621–626

Roach M 3rd, Lu J, Pilepich MV *et al.* (2000). Predicting long-term survival, and the need for hormonal therapy: a meta-analysis of RTOG prostate cancer trials. *International Journal of Radiation Oncology Biology Physics* **47**, 617–627

Ross KS, Carter HB, Pearson JD *et al.* (2000). Comparative efficiency of prostate-specific antigen screening strategies for prostate cancer detection. *Journal of the American Medical Association* **284**, 1399–1405

Rutqvist LE & Wilking N (1992). Analogues of LHRH versus orchidectomy: comparison of economic costs for castration in advanced prostate cancer. *British Journal of Cancer* **65**, 927–929

Stamey TA, Donaldson AN, Yemoto CE *et al.* (1998). Histology and clinical findings in 896 consecutive prostates treated only with radical retropubic prostatectomy: epidemiologic significance of annual changes. *Journal of Urology* **160**, 2412–2417

Wagner TT, Young D, Bahnson R (1999). Charge and length of stay for radical retropubic prostatectomy and transperineal brachytherapy. *Journal of Urology* **161**, 1216–1220

Wilson JMG & Jungner G (1968). *Principles and Practice of Screening for Diseases.* Geneva: WHO

Wolf JS Jr, Cher M, Dall'era M *et al.* (1995). The use and accuracy of cross-sectional imaging and fine needle aspiration cytology for detection of pelvic lymph node metastases before radical prostatectomy. *Journal of Urology* **153**, 993–999

Index